Living With Psychosis

Recovery and Wellbeing

Elina Baker &
Melanie Attwater

chipmunkapublishing
the mental health publisher

Published by
Chipmunkapublishing
United Kingdom

http://www.chipmunkapublishing.com

Copyright © 2015 Elina Baker & Melanie Attwater

ISBN   978-1-78382-231-7

The publication of this book has been funded by Recovery Devon, a community of people of good will, supporting mental health recovery and wellbeing.

To all those who live with psychosis,
as a personal experience or as a supporter to someone else.

With grateful acknowledgments to Glenn Roberts and James Wooldridge for their editorial contributions and championing our vision to help make it a reality.

With thanks to the board of directors of Recovery Devon for their enthusiastic support of the project, especially Elaine Hewis for providing further review of our work.

With special thanks to all the other people who helped to make the Life with Psychosis group (and the families and carers group) a success, through being prepared to share their experiences and offer their wisdom, for the benefit of others: Andy, Annabel, Ashley, Rebecca and Jonny.

'Living with Psychosis: Recovery and Wellbeing'

Contents

Who are we and why are we writing this book?

Elina Baker

I am a clinical psychologist and I have worked with people with psychosis for fifteen years. During this time I have learnt about organisations like the Hearing Voices network and how people with psychosis can help each other move forward from that experience. I have also seen how mental health services can sometimes make things worse for people, through giving them medication with debilitating side effects or making them feel that they have no control over their lives. As a result, I decided to set up groups where people could learn about other ways of coping with their experiences and hear about recovery from people who knew what it was like, because they'd been through it themselves. I was delighted to have the opportunity to work with Melanie, who could bring both her personal perspective and a lot of valuable knowledge from her work as an occupational therapist.

We've seen people learn and grow through coming to the Life with Psychosis group, and then getting involved in running it, sharing the benefit of their experience with people at an earlier stage on the recovery journey. I know that groups can be difficult, especially for people with psychosis, who can feel very wary of other people and get easily overwhelmed. So, I hope that this book will give more people the chance to learn about ways of coping with and understanding their experience of psychosis. It is meant to be a work book that someone can go through on their own, or with the support of a mental health worker. Obviously we can't put in all the information that someone will need so there are lots of suggestions of other places to find out more about the topics we discuss. The book is written in the order we discuss topics in the group, as our group members have found it helpful to develop coping strategies before tackling the challenging questions about how to make sense of their experiences. However, you can look at the different sections in whatever order works for you.

Melanie Attwater

I wanted to help write this book to give hope and motivation to people who have psychosis.

When I had my first psychotic episode twenty years ago all I wanted was for someone to tell me that something good could come out of the situation I found myself in.   Since then I have discovered that psychosis could actually be a blessing. Psychosis has given my life a purpose, a sense of focus and direction and changed me as a person.   My subsequent career in mental health has given me fulfilment, rewards, and a productive role full of personal meaning.

My recovery started by learning everything I could about mental health. I found it to be a fascinating subject. I learnt how to make sense of my own experiences and look for the kernel of truth in all my memories, fears and preoccupations. I needed to know why I had become unwell and more importantly how I could get better and have a good life.

An Occupational Therapist helped me and she seemed a real and reachable person. Also I was envious of her job: it seemed varied and creative. After my Occupational Therapy training I have been working in mental health ever since, now as a Senior Mental Health Practitioner in the Psychosis and Recovery Team.

I now see the same doctors and nurses at my work that have treated me in the past, as I work in the same NHS Trust. I feel no embarrassment. Instead I feel in quite a powerful position to have a patient's view of the people who are also my colleagues. I hope I can remind them that recovery is real and possible and right beside them.

I feel I can help the people with mental health problems that come to me. I treat them in the way I wish I had always been treated, and I share my knowledge of recovery with them to try and give them hope and motivation to find a recovery path for themselves. I try to help them find a positive perspective of their experiences.

I have been co facilitating the Life With Psychosis Group since it began in 2011. In the group I have met many inspiring, intelligent and kind people with psychosis. They are all people who are looking for ways to explore their

7

experiences, to find understanding and holistic wellbeing for themselves and for each other. I hope to share some of the positivity we experience as a group to inspire others that psychosis can be a positive experience and a path to living a full, meaningful and satisfying life.

A note about language

We think that language is important. The words that are used about us and that we use to describe ourselves and our experiences shape our identities and expectations, they let us know who we are and what we can achieve. Unfortunately, the kinds of words that have been used to talk about people who have experienced psychosis have often left them feeling worthless, hopeless, different and excluded. In this book we hope to challenge some of these negative understandings and expectations and so we have tried to use language to reflect our belief that people who experience psychosis are, first and foremost, people. We often hear people describe themselves as 'a schizophrenic' or 'a service user', as if their unusual experiences or mental health are the most important thing about them and the kind of life they can live is set in stone. We also hear people talk about the kind of experiences we describe in this book as symptoms of an illness; we don't think there is any right way to understand these kinds of experiences and we also know that there are other ways of understanding and talking about them that might be more helpful. So we have tried to avoid medical language, because these kinds of experiences happen to a lot of people and could mean all kinds of different things; describing something as an illness often makes people think that its down to doctors to treat with medicines, rather than something they can understand and tackle themselves. It's not easy when mental health services are so full of medical language but we do our best to find ways of talking about the experiences people have that make them seem natural, human and possible to overcome. We also think its better if people can find their own words to describe their experiences, rather than using the words that someone else has given them. This reflects the uniqueness of the person's experience and puts them in control of deciding who they are and what has happened to them.

So, we ask you to take a moment to think about the words that you use to describe yourself:

• Do you ever describe yourself in terms of your diagnosis or as a service user? Could you re-phrase this so that you are a person first? (e.g.: a person who hears voices, a person who uses mental health services?)

• Do you describe your experiences in medical terms? Have you thought about whether this is the best way of describing your experiences? Are there other non-medical words you could use instead (e.g.: talking about experiences rather than symptoms, or distress rather than illness).

• How would you have described your experiences before someone told you they were symptoms of an illness? (e.g.: being in another world, being in fear of your life, being controlled by a mysterious force). Does using your own language make a difference to how you feel about yourself and what happened to you?

Chapter 1: What do we mean by psychosis?

'Psychosis' is a word that is used to describe a range of out of the ordinary experiences, which the other people around you don't share. Some common experiences are:

• hearing voices or other noises that don't seem to come from anywhere
• seeing things or seeing things differently to other people around you
• having strange sensations in your body
• thinking that you are being persecuted or that people are trying to hurt you
• thinking things have special meanings (e.g.: TV and radio broadcasts, car number plates)
• thinking you have special powers (e.g.: being a Messiah, telepathy)
• thinking you are under surveillance, being watched or shown on TV
• thinking that someone is interfering with your thoughts, putting them into you head or taking them away.

These experiences usually seem very real, but because other people around you are not aware of them, we describe them as 'experiences outside of our shared reality'.
There are lots of reasons why people might have these kinds of experiences and we will explore these in later sections of the book. Doctors will often diagnose someone who is troubled by these experiences with a mental illness, such as schizophrenia, schizoaffective disorder or bipolar disorder.

Does it matter which diagnosis I have been given?
A diagnosis is the name given to a group of experiences or difficulties that doctors think reflect a particular underlying medical condition. There is a lot of disagreement about whether the different mental health diagnoses really do reflect different conditions. This is because there is a lot of overlap in the symptoms and someone diagnosed with schizophrenia can have more in common with someone

diagnosed with bipolar disorder than someone else with schizophrenia. People's experiences also change over time so their experiences can seem to reflect different conditions at different times in their life (see Melanie's experiences below). Like Melanie, some people end up being given lots of different diagnoses for these reasons.

Many people don't like having a diagnosis, because they feel that they end up being treated like a label rather than a person. Some people do find it helpful, as it gives them a clear idea about what is wrong with them. We'll discuss the advantages and disadvantages of this more in section eight. We think it is most helpful to look at what experiences someone is actually having (such as hearing voices or feeling paranoid) and think about how to help them cope with that, so we won't talk much about the different diagnoses in this book.

How common are these experiences?

These kinds of experiences are much more common than most people think. There have been lots of different studies, which seem to show that about 15% of all people hear voices, but some studies show that as many as 70-80% of people may hear voices at times of stress or loss (such as after someone has died). Many people also have beliefs that are not based in evidence or shared reality. For example, in a survey, nearly half of people in the UK said that they believed in telepathy. Research has found that 10-15% of people experience believing that someone is persecuting them and in one study, 47% of college students said they had experienced paranoia.

We also know that there are lots of people who have these kinds of experiences and don't need help. In the 1980s the Dutch psychiatrist, Marius Romme wanted to find out more about the experience of hearing voices. He spoke to over 400 people who heard voices and about a third of them didn't use mental health services. They found that these people had ways of coping with their voices or even felt they made their lives better. They learnt that people who coped well usually had a way of making sense of their voices and so were able to accept them. They also felt accepted and supported by the people around them.

This means that having experiences outside of shared reality doesn't have to be a problem. In fact some people are proud of it, or see it as a gift or a blessing. This also means that if you can find ways of understanding, accepting and coping with your experiences, and find other people who accept them too, then you may no longer be so troubled by them.

Melanie's experience of psychosis

Someone in hospital once told me she had an 'overactive imagination and a high level of anxiety'. That sums it up for me too. I was given the diagnosis 'schizophrenia', with mainly positive symptoms, e.g. voices, smells, visions, tactile hallucinations, delusions and persecutory thoughts.

I have been admitted to psychiatric hospital four times. The first time I was a voluntary patient and I learnt how terrifying acute wards are, since then I have tried to resist them. My three subsequent stays in hospital were all under Section 3 of the Mental Health Act. The Approved Mental Health Professionals and Doctors considered my behaviour risky and detrimental to my health. Once I left the house at 3am in my pyjamas and waited in a car park for God to take me away. If this behaviour is risky, then maybe the powers that be have a point. I say maybe because I know that no one can argue with beliefs about God.

I believed my purpose on earth was to save the world from evil, illness and destruction. I thought that I could communicate with aliens and animals, vast populations and their political or religious representatives, all to help me in my mission. I thought I had the cure for AIDS, Cancer, even Mental Illness. Mother Nature was like a person to me, who I felt an imperative to help. Most spiritually I felt like I had a very close relationship with God and He spoke to me. One day I sat for hours in the ward lounge convinced that God was sitting there with me, on another chair. It was an enthralling, enchanting experience, one that I would love to have again.

Sometimes my beliefs were more fearful. I was frightened that people could read my thoughts, as they flashed across my forehead. I had literally no secrets, no mind of my own. I thought the world was all laughing at my biggest embarrassments. I also thought I was going to be killed and it was terrifying.

When I felt my head was literally about to fall apart I tied a scarf around my head to try to hold it together. I would do headstands to try to get my brain back into my skull because I feared it was literally breaking apart, falling down and dropping away from me. Sometimes I would eat strange inedible things because I believed them to be parts of me that needed to be back in my body.

I thought about aliens, witches, past lives, ghosts, demons, angels and reincarnation. I worried about death and the afterlife so much I no longer knew how to live.

Alongside the delusions and hallucinations I also experienced mood changes on my last admission to hospital. The diagnosis was changed from 'schizophrenia' to 'schizoaffective disorder'. When I was high I felt invincible, attractive and powerful. I danced all night listening to the same CD. I did not feel hungry or tired. I wanted to buy and read every newspaper, as everything in them was significant to my life. I gave money away because I felt rich. My humour became caustic and I felt funnier than ever before. I was also extremely irritable and hostile. Like pre -menstrual tension that lasted all month long, with panic attacks and paranoia. I felt like I disagreed with everyone about everything, clearly this was problematic on a ward environment.

On leaving the hospital, having calmed down and apologised, and returned home to my husband; I was struck by a lethargy I had never experienced before. I could not do anything, not leave the house or even make a phone call. I lay down most of the day, once on the living room rug because I couldn't be bothered to climb the stairs and lay on my bed. I neglected to make myself a drink because I didn't feel capable of the task, and the thought of putting my empty finished cup in the dishwasher was more than I could manage. All I could do was to survive and remember... 'This too will pass'... and it did pass eventually.

Section for reflection:

What unusual experiences do you have that other people don't share?

Have you been given a diagnosis? How do you feel about it?

Are there any aspects of your experience which you are glad that you have?

How do you relate to Melanie's experience? Have similar things happened to you?

Chapter 2. Is recovery possible?

The short answer is 'yes'! However, the word recovery is used in two different ways:

Getting 'back to normal'

Although we don't find it helpful to talk about diagnosis, a lot of the research that has been done on people with psychosis has focussed on people who had been given a diagnosis of schizophrenia, so that's what we'll describe here. In the past, doctors used to believe that people with schizophrenia wouldn't get better, that their experiences would never improve and they would never be able to look after themselves. However, research has found that, over periods of many years, the majority of people (50-70%) do 'get back to normal'. Depending on the research, this has meant that they have their own homes, jobs and families, that they no longer use mental health services or take medication.

'Getting back to normal' might not be the best way of thinking about recovery though, as not everyone wants the same things in life and there is no reason why we should all live in the same way.

Life would be pretty boring if we did

Psychosis is also a life changing event, so it would be impossible for someone to go back to being just how they were before it happened.

As one of the family members of a person with psychosis put it in a group:

'You can't step in the same river twice'

(because the water has moved on downstream).

Personal recovery

As well as this research, we know that recovery is possible because some people who have experienced psychosis have shared their stories of recovery. Here are some famous examples (you might like to look them up on the internet to learn more about them):

- **Rufus May**, who was diagnosed with schizophrenia as a teenager but managed to leave the mental health system behind, until he trained as a clinical psychologist and went back to work in it.
- **Ron Coleman**, who describes himself as having spent ten years in the mental health system being made into a 'perfect schizophrenic' but who found a way out through joining a 'hearing voices group' and now runs a successful business providing training and consultancy in mental health.
- **Pat Deegan**, an American psychologist and researcher who was diagnosed with schizophrenia as a teenager and was told that she wouldn't recover but who is now world famous for her work on mental health recovery.

Although these people have become well known, there is nothing particularly special or unique about them. They show what is possible for everybody who experiences psychosis.

On the basis of the experiences of people who have successfully moved forward from psychosis, many people have started to use the word recovery to mean 'living as well as possible'. They have also shown us that recovery is a process, a journey, not a destination. It is about acceptance, of the difficult things in life and learning how to manage them, recognising that there will always be difficulties along the way. One of the people in our groups used this quote from the scientist and meditation teacher Jon Kabat-Zinn to describe this:

'You can't stop the waves, but you can learn to surf'

Researchers (like Pat Deegan) have tried to find common themes or ideas in the stories that people have shared about their process of recovery. These suggest that what helps people move forward with their recovery is:

- Feeling connected to other people
- Finding hope for a better life

- Building a positive identity: seeing yourself as a person, not a diagnosis or a patient
- Making sense of the experience of psychosis and finding meaning in life
- Feeling in control, of your mental health, and your life

We hope that the stories and ideas in this book will help you in working on these areas. People who've experienced recovery have also said that it does require work. There are no 'magic bullets' and while some of the techniques we'll describe sound simple, putting them into practice, over and over again is hard work. James, another person who helped us lead the group, made a helpful comparison. He had some problems with his back and so he was sent to a physiotherapist. They couldn't just give him a treatment that would make him better. Instead they gave him exercises that he would have to repeat every day for several weeks. He said that his mental health recovery was the same: he had to put the effort in and keep practising, in order to build up his mental fitness. It was hard work but it paid off.

As well as the people we've already mentioned there are some other, more famous examples of people who've experienced psychosis and gone on to do remarkable things:

- John Nash: the subject of the film 'A Beautiful Mind', who was diagnosed with paranoid schizophrenia as a young man but went on to win the Nobel prize for economics.
- Brian Wilson: the lead singer of The Beach Boys, who was diagnosed with schizoaffective disorder in the 1960s but who came back to continue recording and performing sell out concerts.
- Carrie Fisher: the actress who played Princess Leia in Star Wars and who was diagnosed with bipolar disorder but who continues to be an award winning actress and screenwriter

There are also lots of collections of stories about recovery written by people with psychosis. You might like to look at:

In print

Psychosis: Stories of Recovery and Hope (2011), Hannah Cordle, Jane Fradgely, Jerome Carson, Frank Holloway & Paul Richards: Quay Books.

Living with Voices: 50 Stories of Recovery (2009) Marius Romme, Sandra Escher, Jacqui Dillon, Dirk Corstens & Mervyn Morris: PCCS Books

Voicing Psychotic Experiences (2009), Ruth Chandler & Mark Hayward: OLM-Pavilion

Available online for free download

Beyond the Storms: Reflections on Personal Recovery in Devon
http://www.recoverydevon.co.uk/download/Beyond_the_Storms.pdf

Journeys of Recovery: Scottish Recovery Network
http://www.scottishrecovery.net/View-document/81-Journeys-of-Recovery.html?format=raw&tmpl=component

"Kia Mauri Tau" - Narratives of Recovery from Disabling Mental Health Problems: Report of the University of Waikato mental health narratives project
http://www.recoverydevon.co.uk/download/Kia_Mauri_Tau.pdf

Melanie's experience of recovery

The first step towards recovery for me has always been the right medication. I do not like it but I rely on the tablets to recognise myself and the world around me. Each time I have stopped taking the medication I have become acutely psychotic and not able to remain at home, even with the Crisis Team visiting me twice a day. But recovery is more than just taking a tablet. It is about finding out how to help yourself, rediscovering your life and trying to make it habitable again.

Each time I have been admitted to hospital my mental health deteriorated further, into bizarre craziness. Each time I have hit rock bottom, and only then started the arduous ascent back to being me. It's a long way to climb back up when you have been pinned to the floor, and injected against your will, struggling every inch of the way. Enforced injections have to be the quickest way to humiliate and frighten someone. Sometimes it surprises me that I have survived, and even thrived afterwards.

After each acute psychotic episode it has felt like I am starting all over again, I have to regain my confidence and rebuild my life. It takes courage, trust and persistence.

I have had a few people, both family and friends alongside me each time and these people have given me the strength to persist. They have shown me love, patience and understanding; without them I do not think I would have wanted to return to reality. And it does seem like a choice, like weighing up two different worlds and deciding to live in the real world, with everyone else, because it has more to offer. But it still feels like I'm taking a leap of faith. My imaginary world can have things to offer too. Also while I'm in hospital my real life responsibilities narrow right down to having enough cigarettes. It can be an escape from real life and can feel like a holiday from all the confines of normal stresses.

In essence having a life to come back to is what really matters. I am lucky to have a supportive family and friends and I feel blessed beyond anything to have met my husband who has provided me with ceaseless love and loyalty for fourteen years.

It has been important for me to discover what works best for me. We have a lovely home that we share with our cat. Animals make me smile and stop, take time to be in the moment. My favourite hobby is swimming and I can go to the pool when I need to rebalance physically and emotionally. I can walk along the river, and appreciate the fresh air and a fresh perspective. I spend quality time with my friends, and I speak to my Mum every day. I aim to sleep uninterrupted for 9 hours each night. My husband cooks me healthy homemade food. I also have my faith and although my beliefs may seem strange to conventionally religious people, it means I always have something to turn to when needed.

It is not particularly restful thinking about what I need in my life and what I need to avoid at any moment, but it seems necessary to make deliberate choices that keep me on the recovery path. When I have unusual experiences which still happens, like voices or finding special meaning in everyday things, I try to use these times as a wake-up call for what I'm lacking; usually time and space to be quiet and rest and reflect on whatever is upsetting my emotional balance. I see the experiences as lessons for me to learn. I am a person that has a serious mental health problem/sensitivity and I am managing to live a full life at the same time.

My recovery motto is a quote by Rumi, 'to live life as if everything is rigged in your favour'. Sometimes when I sit and try to be mindful I know that all is well. Recovery is reachable and within grasp of everyone but it does take effort and thinking yourself lucky.

Section for reflection:

What does living as well as possible mean to you?

Look at some recovery stories written by other people who have experienced psychosis: what can you learn from them?

What have you already learned about what you need to do to look after yourself?

Chapter 3. Learning to manage your feelings

In chapter one, we mentioned that lots of people have unusual thoughts and experiences but do not feel the need to seek help from mental health services. This suggests that what makes these experiences a problem is how we react to them and our feelings about them. So, learning to manage your feelings is a good place to start in having more control over your mental health.

As we saw in Melanie's description of her experience, psychosis can lead to lots of different distressing or difficult feelings:

- Fear: of coming to harm from voices or persecution.
- Anger: at being treated unfairly, by voices, people persecuting you or even people around you who are trying to help, because they don't believe you.
- Sadness and despair: through feeling people dislike you or want to hurt you, or feeling trapped and alone with your experience
- Over-excited and energetic: if your experiences make you feel special or that you have exciting new knowledge. Although this feels good it can often lead to burn-out or conflict with other people.

A way of understanding distress

We can think of our reactions to what happens to us as being made up of four parts, which all affect each other: thoughts, emotional feelings, physical feelings and behaviour or actions (this is the model used in Cognitive Behaviour Therapy or CBT):

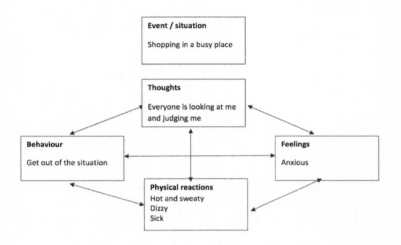

When something happens to us, we will have **_thoughts_** about it, and they will affect how we feel. Here's a simple example:

Imagine you are alone in your house late at night. You hear a noise in another part of the house: What do you think? How would that make you feel? What do you do? Now, try to think of another possible explanation and see if that makes a difference to how you'd feel and what you'd do.

Event	Thoughts	Feelings	Behaviour
Hear noise late at night			

Here's an example from one of our groups:

Event	Thoughts	Feelings	Behaviour
	It's a burglar	Scared	Call the police
Hear noise late at night	It's my friend wanting to see me	Angry at being disturbed	Shout at him to go away
	It's my cat	Relieved that the cat is home	Go back to sleep

This means we can change our feelings by changing our thoughts about a situation. Looking at the example in the diagram above, if your thoughts were 'no one's looking at me, they're all too busy getting on with their shopping', you'd feel much calmer and able to carry on with your own shopping.

There are **physical reactions in our body** that go along with different feelings. The one we'll talk about most is the 'flight or fight' reaction that happens when we are scared, angry or excited. These are some of the common signs:

- Heart races or skips a beat
- Chest feels tight, breathing quickly
- Stomach churning, feeling sick or having 'butterflies'
- Muscles feel tense or body aches
- Feel dizzy or light headed
- Need to go to the toilet
- Sweating
- Vision may narrow or become sharper and hearing may be more sensitive
- Feel jumpy or restless

This is your body's natural response to you feeling under threat: it is getting ready to fight danger or to run away from it. Your body doesn't know if you are actually under threat, or if you just think you are, so if our thoughts about a situation make us feel frightened, this will set the 'flight or fight' reaction going. Unfortunately, it also makes our thoughts focus more on possible threats, keeping our emotional response going.

If most people feel like running away, then that's what they'll do. So, often when we feel frightened we get out of the situation and try and avoid going back into it. Unfortunately, this means that we don't get the chance to find out that we may have misunderstood the situation, or that we can cope with it. So, our thoughts and feelings affect our **behaviour**, which in turns affects our thoughts and feelings, meaning we go on being scared or upset about something when we don't need to.

We'll talk in more detail about how this applies to voices and other unusual experiences and ideas in later chapterss of the book. For now we're going to look at some ways of managing your thoughts, feelings and behaviours in relation to any situation, so that they don't get out of control and cause problems.

Challenging your thoughts

Try and notice your thoughts about situations that you are finding distressing and try to find another way of thinking about the situation:

- Is there another way of looking at it?

- Is your thought true? Is it an opinion or a fact? How do you know?

- What would someone else that you respect think in this situation?

- Is my reaction in proportion to the actual event?

Relaxation exercises

Using a quick breathing exercise can help manage fear and anger by shutting down the 'fight or flight' reaction. Try these two exercises, which people in the group have found helpful:

Seven-Eleven breathing

Making an out-breath last longer than an in-breath can switch on your body's natural relaxation system. As you breathe in, count from one to seven. As you breathe out, count from one to eleven. The counting will also help to distract you from whatever you are worried about.

Diaphragmatic breathing

Sit or lie in a comfortable position. Place your hands palm down on your stomach at the base of the rib cage, middle fingers barely touching each other, and take a slow deep breath. As your lungs completely fill, the diaphragm pushes down and the stomach will slightly expand causing the fingertips to separate. As you breathe out your fingertips will come together again. Try to practice doing this for at least five minutes.

Self-soothing

It can be helpful to have strategies to help you feel calm, comforted and cared for when you feel distressed and overwhelmed, so that you stay in control and do not act on

your feelings. The idea of 'self- soothing' comes from Dialectical Behaviour Therapy (or DBT). A helpful way of remembering what to do is to think of how you can sooth each of your five senses:
Vision
Hearing
Smell
Taste
Touch

Here are some of our favourite examples:

Vision: go outside and walk in nature, visit your favourite view, look at your favourite paintings in a book or online, buy yourself some flowers.
Hearing: play classical music, go out and listen to birdsong, listen to the waves crashing on the beach, listen to children playing
Smell: light a scented candle, use a scented hand cream, smell some flowers, smell the bread baking in a shop, walk in the woods or on the beach and breathe deeply
Taste: have a hot chocolate or herbal tea, cook your favourite meal or try a new recipe.
Touch: have a bath, stroke a pet, cuddle a teddy bear, wrap yourself in a blanket, go for a swim.

'Opposite to emotion' action

This idea is also from Dialectical Behaviour Therapy and like all the ideas, it sounds simple but it is not easy to put into practice and can take effort and persistence. It simply means doing the opposite of how you feel. So, if you feel angry and want to lash out, using that anger to walk away and do something useful or kind. If you feel sad, don't stay in bed but go out and do something you usually enjoy. If you feel scared, don't hide away but keep going out, carrying on with your usual routine.
Starting by changing your behaviour can make a difference to how you are thinking and how you are feeling and so take you out of the difficult reaction.

Unhelpful ways of coping with feelings

Sometimes people find ways of managing their difficult feelings that are harmful or end up making the problem worse. Some common examples are:

- Taking street drugs, like cannabis, speed, Ecstasy, heroin or cocaine
- Using legal highs
- Drinking alcohol
- Self harming

We know that these strategies can help people feel better in the short term, making them feel happier or less tense, sometimes blocking their experiences out. However, they often have negative consequences in the longer term, so the withdrawal effects from drugs and alcohol can make psychosis worse and people can feel very ashamed of self-harming, not to mention the damaging effect of all these strategies on your body. Although there is still some debate about whether and how taking drugs might cause psychosis, they do have a powerful effect on your mind and your sense of reality (which is why people take them!) and many people find that they contribute to their experiences in some way. For some drugs (e.g.: speed, alcohol), this might be while you're withdrawing or coming down from them, rather then when you're actually using them, as this can have a powerful effect on our emotions too.

If you are using any of these ways of coping, it can be helpful to really think through all the advantages and disadvantages and see if it might be making things worse for you overall. You could also think through the advantages and disadvantages of the other strategies we've suggested. We use the format on the next page to help people do this and we've filled in some examples for someone who is drinking alcohol:

Pros (benefits) of using this strategy	Cons (costs) of using this strategy
Feel more relaxed Feel happier Block voices out More confident and sociable Something to do with friends	Hangover- waste next day in bed Feel paranoid Voices worse next day Say stupid things & hurt people's feelings Spend too much money Mum doesn't like it Gaining weight Need to drink more to get the same effect
Pros (benefits) of using a self-soothing strategy instead	Cons (costs) of using a self-soothing strategy instead
Feel in control of behaviour Feel good about myself Feel healthier People are proud of me Cheaper than drinking Gets easier with practice	Doesn't block things out as quickly Have to put more effort in

In thinking about the costs and benefits of the strategy it can be helpful to think about how it affects:

- Your health and wellbeing (physically and mentally)
- Your relationships with family, partners and friends
- Your work or studies and financial situation
- How you fit in to society (does it get you in trouble or make you more likely to be sectioned?)

Its also helpful to think about both the immediate and longer term effects, as these strategies can often make you feel better straight away but end up causing harm.

Melanie's experience

Everyone has difficult feelings and has to find ways of coping with them. I believe in Maya Angelou's quote, 'When you know better you do better.' Before I had any contact with mental health services I used to smoke cannabis to help me sleep and drank alcohol to make myself relax. These were coping strategies that I used at that time, but they made me feel worse. They may work in the short term, but ultimately lead to more problems.

Sometimes I still feel very overwhelmed by negative feelings, it feels like a constant struggle to relax and return to the landscape of normality. Sometimes I feel my negative, tense feelings go on for so long it is like they have become my new normal baseline. But there are always things I can do about it, there are always ways I can help myself. Even getting out of bed can be a challenge some days when I just want to hide away and try to sleep. But having a job gives me routine and structure and a good reason not to stay in bed all day. Working in mental health can be emotionally draining so I need to find people and activities that replenish my resources and give me comfort.

When I feel the stress of living in the real world and coping with the rat race becomes too much for me I will take a day off work and try to find ways to recuperate and rebalance. I make sure I have a shower and get dressed and then I go for a walk and I will call my mum. I will read a good book or a watch a film to escape or drown out negative feeling by eating something sweet and filling. I will try to write about my feelings in my journal. I try to breathe deeply and slowly and sometimes Rescue remedy or lavender oil will relax me. Often I will go for a swim as this always helps or I will take the time to care for myself and my appearance. At night I will have warm bath as this helps me get a good long night sleep, the next day, as if restored, I carry on as normal.

When I talk to my colleagues about feeling stressed I realise that we can all have bad feelings and difficult demands on us, it is normal and human to have stress, and it is not unusual for mental health staff to find it difficult to cope sometimes. Maybe the voice shouting in my head makes my challenge unusual and maybe I need more time to think through how to respond in ways that won't alienate me. My biggest challenge is learning how not to pass on the bad feelings to other people. When the voice shouts at me and tells me what to do I reciprocate by seeming rude and irrational to others and this behaviour may seem unreasonable but I think it is an understandable response to what is happening inside.

My medication helps by making my feelings blunted and easier to live with. I endeavour to take them every day and learn from the times that I have come off the tablets. The medication however is not the only answer, it cannot make me feel authentic and self knowing, but the other self-soothing things can do this.

Psychosis has made me even more aware of what I need to do to look after myself. Recovery is about making yourself do the things that you know will help.

Section for reflection:

Try and use the diagram below to explore how the thoughts, feelings and behaviours you have in response to stressful or upsetting events: Can you see how they affect each other?

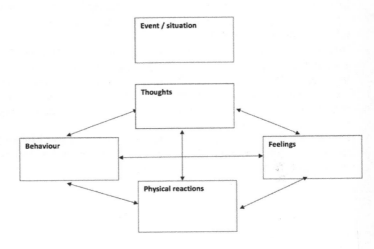

Try some of the strategies we describe to change your feelings and behaviours: Do they make a difference?

Do you have any of coping strategies which may be harmful in the longer term? What are the advantages and disadvantages for you of using these strategies? What could you do instead?

Chapter 4. Using mindfulness to manage thoughts and feelings

Mindfulness began over 2000 years ago as a Buddhist meditation practice but it is now widely used by people of all faiths (and none) as a tool to help manage stress and it has been shown to improve mental health. A simple definition of mindfulness is:

'Paying attention in a particular way, on purpose, in the present moment and non-judgmentally'
Or, in other words, focussing your mind on the things that are happening to you *right now* and trying to just notice what you are experiencing, rather than reacting to it. Here's how this can be helpful:

Think about some things that upset you. Are they:

- Memories of difficult things that have happened in the past?
- Worries about what you think will happen in the future?

These are what upset most people and so we think that learning to pay attention to just the present moment is helpful as it allows us to let go of difficult thoughts and feelings. It also means we can appreciate things around us that we don't normally notice because we are caught up in our memories, plans and worries.
Try the raisin exercise at the end of this chapter (it's usually done with a raisin but you could use other small food items such as grapes or sweets). The point of the exercise is to get you to focus on your immediate experience of something, noticing your responses to it and how letting go of them can change the way you experience something very ordinary. It will work best if you read it through, so you know what you need to do, then try and do it. It's even better if you can get someone else to read it to you, or you can look it up on You Tube so you can listen to it.

What did you notice while you were doing this exercise? Most people find that they get distracted by their thoughts and have to keep bringing their attention back to the raisin. This can be frustrating but it is how you learn the skill of mindfulness, by continuously noticing that your mind has wandered and bringing it back to noticing your immediate experience. People also say that it's the best raisin they've ever tasted, because they've taken the time to really notice it!

We can take a mindful approach to anything we do (eating, walking, washing up etc.) but it can be helpful to take some time out regularly to do a mindfulness practice, as it helps us to be more aware of our thoughts and feelings, and learn to let go of them. This skill then carries over into our everyday life, meaning that we are more able to go into situations calmly and manage our reactions capably. In trying to be mindful, it helps to have an anchor: something that you can keep bringing your attention back to. We suggest that people use their breathing, as this is something you always have with you. Try the mindful breathing exercise at the end of the chapter (again, you can listen to it online)

From trying this exercise, you should be able to discover that your thoughts and feelings come and go: you can't help having them but you can allow them to pass, rather than getting caught up in them or overwhelmed by them

Developing a mindful response to psychosis

Mindfulness can be a helpful way of managing our emotional responses to all kinds of situations. People can find it particularly hard to put into practice when it comes to psychosis though, as these experiences can feel very frightening and overwhelming. Mindfulness can feel like letting go of control over your mind and when something terrifying is trying to get in, that's the last thing you want to do. So in this chapter we'll explore a bit more how letting go, and accepting, psychosis can actually help you be more in control.

Think about what your experiences are (voices, visions, strange sensations, disturbing thoughts). Now make a list of how you respond. Next, think about any advantages and disadvantages. Often people find that their responses make things better in the short term but make things worse in the longer term. We've put in some examples to show what we mean;

Response	Advantages	Disadvantages
Playing music loudly to drown out voices	Don't listen to voices as much	Don't hear phone ringing Voices get louder
Writing down everything that happens to prove what is going on	Feel like I'm taking positive action	People don't take it seriously or get angry Forget to cook dinner because I'm too busy writing
Have a drink	Blocks voices out	Hangover and feel worse the next day Voices criticise me for drinking too much

Most responses that people come up with can be divided up into two categories:
- avoiding or blocking out the experience (eg by distracting yourself or drowning it out)
- getting lost or caught up in the experience (eg by paying attention to it, trying to think of ways out of it)

Both of these types of response have disadvantages: either you to have work really hard at keeping your experiences out of your mind (which can be exhausting or damage your health, if you use strategies like drink or drugs) or you get so pre-occupied with the experience that you can't do anything else and may even stop taking proper care of yourself.

Mindfulness is a middle way between these two types of response. A mindful response is to notice that the experience is there, accepting and observing it but not reacting to it or acting on it, just allowing it to come and go again.

We know that this is easier said than done, especially when the things you see, hear and think make you feel very frightened. Remember how when you tried the 'mindfulness of breath' exercise, you were able to notice thoughts and sensations and then bring your attention back to your breath? It is possible to just notice all thoughts and sensations, even ones that can seem alarming, in the same way, without getting caught up in worrying about them or trying to understand them.

It can help to think of all your experiences, and thoughts and feelings about them as being like a waterfall, coming down on your head. You can take a step back, so that you are behind the waterfall, watching what is happening, without being part of them, letting them fall past you and disappear.

Another useful guide to help you respond mindfully to difficult experiences and emotions is the RAIN acronym:

- **R – Recognise** the experience you're having or the emotion you're feeling. Name it in your mind if you can.
- **A – Accept** the experience you're having. You might not like the experience or the feeling, but the reality is, it is here at the moment.
- **I – Investigate**. Become curious about your experience. If there are voices, what do they sound like? Where do you feel your emotional response in your body? What kind of thoughts are going through your mind? How are they following on from each other?
- **N – Non-identification.** See the experience as a passing event rather than having any meaning about who you are. Remember thoughts and feelings are beyond your control and come and go.

Try the body scan exercise at the end of the chapter: While you are doing it, if you are interrupted by voices, strange sensations or frightening thoughts, try just to notice and accept that they are there, without getting caught up in thinking about them and bring your attention back to the part of your body you are focusing on. Each time you do so is a moment of mindfulness. Again, if you search for this online you will find sites where you can listen to it.

It is important to remember that mindfulness requires practice and that we may need to bring our attention back to our focus many, many times. The more you practice it though, the easier it will become. The mind is like a muscle and it can be strengthened by training in the same way. So, doing a short mindfulness practice every day can mean that when things get tough, we are ready and can allow even frightening and upsetting things to come and go, noticing, accepting, observing and bring our attention away from them again. As with physical exercise, you will get more benefit from these practices if you do a little but often rather than doing a big burst, finding it too hard and giving up! With regular practice, it can become a useful part of your daily routine.

Melanie's experience

Mindfulness is a form of meditation and can be the most relaxing and regenerating of activities, while doing nothing. A quote by Franz Kafka describes meditation in the most beautiful way:

'You need not leave your room. Remain sitting at your table and listen. You need not even listen, simply wait. You need not even wait, just learn to become quiet, and still, and solitary. The world will freely offer itself to you to be unmasked. It has no choice. It will roll in ecstasy at your feet.'

I started my mindfulness practice by listening to a CD with guiding instructions. I never became particularly disciplined in making a regular time for meditation but I have learnt to incorporate mindfulness in my everyday life, to take time to breathe and witness my thoughts come and go. I find it easiest to use breathing as my anchor when I practice mindfulness. As I focus on my breath it naturally deepens and slows down. A full conscious breath, filling my lungs with air and releasing the breath slowly calms my body and mind. It is in this way that I feel the effects of mediation and I find it deeply relaxing. I am not unique in feeling this benefit, it can work for anybody.

It takes practice and it's important to remember that no one has perfect focus. My mind will jump all over the place and it is challenging not to get carried away with my thinking. Practice has helped me and gradually I find it easier to detach from troublesome thoughts, feelings and voices.

Like other people with psychosis I often search for calming and soothing experiences that can offer space to be mindful between the thoughts, hallucinations and patterns of behaviour that perpetuate negative feelings. I am lucky to live near the coast so I can find respite walking on the beach or sitting in the shade of the trees. Being with my cat also creates mindful moments that prompt me to stay in the present. Likewise when I spend time with my young nieces and nephews it is easy not to think too much, children have such immediate demands that they can help us learn to live in the present.

I have found mindfulness to be a useful strategy for dealing with voices, it seems to stop time and creates a distance between me and my mind's chatter. Difficult thoughts, feelings and hallucinations come into my mind but they also go again. Mindfulness makes me more aware of these things passing.

Section for reflection:

Try the mindfulness exercises: did you notice how you have little control of your thoughts? Did you find that you can allow thoughts to come and go from your mind by changing the focus of your attention?

Did you experience any voices, visions or frightening ideas? Were you able to mentally take a step back from them, noticing and accepting them but also allowing them to come and go?

The raisin exercise

Focus on the objects and just imagine that you have never seen anything like it before. Imagine you have just dropped in from Mars this moment and you have never seen anything like it before in your life.

Take the objects and holding it in the palm of your hand, or between your finger and thumb, pay attention to seeing it. Look at it carefully, as if you had never seen such a thing before. Turn it over between your fingers.

Explore its texture between your fingers. Examine the highlights where the light shines, the darker hollows and folds. Let your eyes explore every part of it, as if you had never seen such a thing before.

If, while you are doing this any thoughts come to mind about "what a strange thing I am doing" or "what is the point of this" or "I don't like these," then just note them as thoughts and bring your awareness back to the object.

Now smell the object, taking it and holding it beneath your nose, and with each in-breath, carefully notice the smell of it.

Now take another look at it.

Now slowly take the object to your mouth, maybe noticing how your hand and arm know exactly where to put it, perhaps noticing your mouth watering as it comes up.

Gently place the object in the mouth, noticing how it is "received" without biting it, just exploring the sensations of having it in your mouth.

When you are ready, very consciously take a bite into it and notice the tastesthat it releases.

Slowly chew it, noticing the saliva in the mouth and the change in consistency of the object.

Then, when you feel ready to swallow, see if you can first detect the intention to swallow as it comes up, so that even this is experienced consciously before you actually swallow it.

Finally, see if you can follow the sensations of swallowing it, sensing it moving down to your stomach, and also realizing that your body is now exactly one raisin heavier.

Mindful breathing

The main goal of mindful breathing is simply a calm, non judging awareness, allowing thoughts and feelings to come and go without getting caught up in them

Sit comfortably, with your eyes closed and your back comfortably straight

Bring your attention to your breathing

Imagine that you have a balloon in your stomach. Every time you breathe in, the balloon inflates. Each time you breathe out, the balloon deflates. Notice the sensations in your stomach as the balloon inflates and deflates. Notice your stomach rising with the in breath...and falling on the out breath.

Thoughts, images and voices may come into your mind. That's ok, because that's what the human mind does. Simply take note without reacting to them, and then return your attention to your breathing.

You don't have to follow those thoughts or feelings, don't judge yourself having them, or analyse them in any way. It's ok for your thoughts to be there. Notice them, and let them drift on like leaves floating down a river. Return to your next breath, in.. and out.

Whenever you find your attention drifting off, notice it, and then return to the sensations and rhythm of your body , and notice how the breath feels in ..and out.. how regular it is.

Really focus on the gentle rhythm of your breathing, if your breath is hot or cold, and how your chest and stomach might move.

When your thoughts wander...keep coming back to your breathing..

When you are ready open your eyes and sit restfully for a moment.

Body Scan Mindfulness Exercise

1. Sit in a chair as for the breath awareness or lie down, making yourself comfortable, lying on your back on a mat or rug on the floor or on your bed. Choose a place where you will be warm and undisturbed. Allow your eyes to close gently.

2. Take a few moments to get in touch with the movement of your breath and the sensations in the body. When you are ready, bring your awareness to the physical sensations in your body, especially to the sensations of touch or pressure, where your body makes contact with the chair or bed. On each outbreath, allow yourself to let go, to sink a little deeper into the chair or bed.

3. Remind yourself of the intention of this practice. Its aim is not to feel any different, relaxed, or calm; this may happen or it may not. Instead, the intention of the practice is, as best you can, to bring awareness to any sensations you detect, as you focus your attention on each part of the body in turn.

4. Now bring your awareness to the physical sensations in the lower abdomen, becoming aware of the changing patterns of sensations in the abdominal wall as you breathe in, and as you breathe out. Take a few minutes to feel the sensations as you breathe in and as you breathe out.

5. Having connected with the sensations in the abdomen, bring the focus or "spotlight" of your awareness down the left leg, into the left foot, and out to the toes of the left foot. Focus on each of the toes of the left foot in turn, bringing a gentle curiosity to investigate the quality of the sensations you find, perhaps noticing the sense of contact between the toes, a sense of tingling, warmth, or no particular sensation.

6. When you are ready, on an inbreath, feel or imagine the breath entering the lungs, and then passing down into the abdomen, into the left leg, the left foot, and out to the toes of the left foot. Then, on the outbreath, feel or imagine the breath coming all the way back up, out of the foot, into the leg, up through the abdomen, chest, and out through the nose. As best you can, continue this for a few breaths, breathing down into the toes, and back out from the toes. It

may be difficult to get the hang of this just practice this "breathing into" as best you can, approaching it playfully.

7. Now, when you are ready, on an outbreath, let go of awareness of the toes, and bring your awareness to the sensations on the bottom of your left foot—bringing a gentle, investigative awareness to the sole of the foot, the instep, the heel (e.g., noticing the sensations where the heel makes contact with the mat or bed). Experiment with "breathing with" the sensations—being aware of the breath in the background, as, in the foreground, you explore the sensations of the lower foot.

8. Now allow the awareness to expand into the rest of the foot—to the ankle, the top of the foot, and right into the bones and joints. Then, taking a slightly deeper breath, directing it down into the whole of the left foot, and, as the breath lets go on the outbreath, let go of the left foot completely, allowing the focus of awareness to move into the lower left leg—the calf, shin, knee, and so on, in turn.

9. Continue to bring awareness, and a gentle curiosity, to the physical sensations in each part of the rest of the body in turn - to the upper left leg, the right toes, right foot, right leg, pelvic area, back, abdomen, chest, fingers, hands, arms, shoulders, neck, head, and face. In each area, as best you can, bring the same detailed level of awareness and gentle curiosity to the bodily sensations present. As you leave each major area, "breathe in" to it on the inbreath, and let go of that region on the outbreath.

10. When you become aware of tension, or of other intense sensations in a particular part of the body, you can "breathe in" to them—using the inbreath gently to bring awareness right into the sensations, and, as best you can, have a sense of their letting go, or releasing, on the outbreath.

11. The mind will inevitably wander away from the breath and the body from time to time. That is entirely normal. It is what minds do. When you notice it, gently acknowledge it, noticing where the mind has gone off to, and then gently return your attention to the part of the body you intended to focus on.

12. After you have "scanned" the whole body in this way, spend a few minutes being aware of a sense of the body as a whole, and of the breath flowing freely in and out of the body.

Chapter 5. Changing your response to voices

In chapter three, we looked at how our responses to events can be thought of as being made up of thoughts, feelings, physical reactions and behaviour. We can also think about our reactions to voices in the same way. Here is an example:

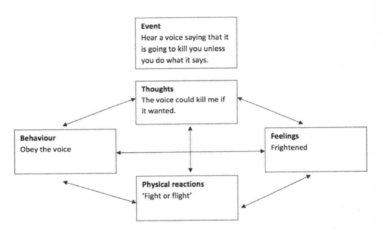

In order to cope with the voice, you could work on any part of your response to it. So, you could use mindfulness to notice and let go of your thoughts and feelings, so you don't react to the voice. Or you could use one of the breathing techniques to calm yourself down so you can think more clearly. This could help you remember that if you try and escape the situation, by doing what the voice wants, you won't find out whether or not the voice can actually carry out its threat to kill you. In this chapter we'll be looking in more depth at how to challenge your thoughts and beliefs about voices.

Common traits of problematic voices

As we've said, not all voices cause people problems. Some voices can be a positive experience and can be kind and helpful. Some people experience both positive and negative voices and some people find that the same voice can be positive and negative at different times. We have found that the voices that cause people problems act like bullies and people usually feel that the voices are more powerful than them.

So, in coping with your voices, it can help to remember what you might have been told about bullies:

- The best way of dealing with bullies is by standing up to them
- Bullies are often frightened and hurt themselves

Like bullies, voices can also be manipulative. They will try to make you feel small and will pick on your weak spots. They often make things up, about you and other people, to make you feel more alone and they often make empty threats, which they can't carry though, so that you will do what they want.

So, our thoughts about problematic voices are often that they are powerful, that they are right about us and that we have to do what they say. But, just as we were able to come up with different explanations for hearing a noise in the house at night, we can come up with different explanations for what voices say:

Event	Thoughts	Feelings	Behaviour
Hear a voice saying that everyone hates you	It must be true, everyone does hate me	Upset	Stay home and don't talk to anyone
	The voice just wants to make me feel bad	Determined	Go out with friends
	The voice must feel pretty bad about itself	Sorry for the voice	Go out with friends

It can help to look for evidence to see whether a voice is telling the truth or not. So if a voice tells you that are useless, you could make a list of all the things that you have done well. Sometimes you can find ways of testing out whether what the voice say is true. If a voice claims to be able to make something happen, you can ask it to prove this by doing it. If they say they can do something dangerous or that you are very scared of, you can ask them to do something smaller. So, if a voice says it can get a car to run you over you might ask it if it can make a pencil roll across the table. If it can't do a small thing, it follows that it can't do a big thing. It can be helpful to ask someone you trust to help you with this, so that you have a witness or a different perspective on the situation. Make sure you are clear about exactly when you want the voice to do something, as voices can take credit for random things which they haven't really caused.

Being assertive

Discovering that voices can't carry out their threats could help you to feel more confident about standing up to them. When responding to voices, its helpful to try and *be assertive*. This means expressing your opinions and saying what you want while also showing respect for the other person's opinions and taking into account what they want. Becoming angry and being aggressive, by shouting and swearing is likely to just make the voices feel threatened and retaliate. Remember that voices may be treating you badly because they are frightened and hurt themselves, so it is important to try and be kind to them. Try saying things which acknowledge the voice's opinion as well as expressing your own feelings and opinions. For example:

"Thank you for your opinion but I disagree".

"I know you don't like it but I don't think there's anything wrong with what I'm doing"

"I can tell that you are angry but it hurts my feelings when you say that, so I want you to stop".

"I can see that you don't like that, but I do"

It can also be helpful to set boundaries, for example by setting a time during the day when it is convenient for the voices to talk to you. This can let the voices know that respect them wanting to talk to you but they need to respect when you want to listen. You may be able to agree other compromises between what the voices want and what you want to.

Listening to voices

Although we cannot be sure where voices come from, they do seem to pick up on and express people's feelings, particularly if they are not expressing these feelings themselves. So, it can be helpful to try and listen to the voices and see what messages they might have for you, For example, if a voice is angry, it may be reflecting something that you are angry about. If a voice is frightening or wants you to hurt yourself, this may reflect that you are feeling frightened or hurt. It can be helpful to try finding ways to express feelings safely, perhaps by writing them down or talking to someone you trust about them. You can also try and reassure and comfort voices, so that they no longer feel the need to make you aware of fear and pain.

Melanie's experience

I began to hear a male voice about a year after my first psychotic episode. It started by giving me instructions over and over again, it seemed to be outside of my head but it was always shouting. The experience was strange and it made me feel very odd and different to begin with.

At first the voice was quite benign, saying things like 'leave England', and I thought that it was helping me.

The voice later became nasty and repeated words like 'kill yourself'. I became distressed and eventually I started to talk about it and this helped me to give the voice that I heard a face and a name that I could relate to. I thought of the voice as one of my relatives who had behaved in threatening and aggressive ways towards me when I was chaotic with psychosis.

I tried to fight the voice and to overpower it but this did not help. Then a few years ago when I had the opportunity I found a brave and effective way to shift the balance of power in my favour. I told my relative that I heard his voice in my head and it was very annoying. I finally felt like I had taken control of the situation. For me it was a turning point. I asserted my opinion and spoke out about how he was making me feel.

As time went by I noticed a new brief moment of consciousness, a small moment of opportunity when I actually listened for the voice before I heard it; instead of just hearing it out of the blue. That split second was enough, I realised I could dictate what the voice would say. In the briefest moment I could change my thoughts and change the content of the voice to make it say things that were more positive. The voice seems to echo my thoughts so I deliberately changed my thoughts. This was a revelation to me. I could actually make the voice say anything I wanted to hear, so I made it say kinder things.

I could make the voice say 'love yourself', instead of 'kill yourself', and so on. I was no longer afraid of it. I have learnt how to be stand up and be respected by the voice in my head and also how to put it to one side. I have learnt that I am in control and not the other way around, and now I 'listen' to than just 'hear' it. Choosing to listen gives me choice and control back.

The voice can seem like company to me. It has been part of my life for twenty years. It is compelling in one way, a companion and someone who always knows what is going on in my head at any moment. It can stop me feeling small as the voice shouts high in the air and makes itself heard. It has become more of a friend to me now, and I think I would miss it, if it I could no longer hear it.

Generally I distract myself by focussing on other more tangible things in my life. I see this process as creating new neural pathways in my mind, new networks that stop me going over the same voice hearing path time and time again. As life is busy and full of other things to focus on the voice is less frequent now, sometimes days or even weeks will pass when I do not hear the voice at all, and I am too busy getting on with my life to even notice.

Other helpful sources of information

If you are interested in finding out more about the way that other people have gained control over their voices, you could look at this book:

Living with Voices: 50 Stories of Recovery by Marius Romme and others. Published by PCCS Books.

Eleanor Longden, whose story is in the book, has also done a talk for TED about her experiences:
http://www.ted.com/talks/eleanor_longden_the_voices_in_m y_head?language=en

There is lots of useful advice about ways of getting control and communicating with voices on Rufus May's website: www.rufusmay.com

Section for reflection:

When you hear a voice what are your thoughts, feelings, physical reactions and behaviours? How could you change them?

Are there ways you could start to stand up to or disagree with your voices? What would an assertive response to your voices be?

Does your voice threaten to do things? How could you test whether it can carry out these threats?

What feelings might your voices be trying to communicate to you about? Can you relate to these feelings? How would like someone to respond to you if you felt that way? Can you give your voices this response?

Chapter 6. Managing worries about conspiracies, paranoia and other troubling unusual ideas and beliefs

In this chapter, we will be talking about ways of coping with what psychiatrists call 'delusions'. Most people hold strong irrational beliefs of one kind or another, so we don't find it helpful to think that there's something fundamentally different about the kind of beliefs that get labelled delusions, and we just think of them as 'unusual beliefs'. We have also met lots of people for whom what is happening to them is not just a belief but, as far as they are concerned, a real experience. We believe that are there many things that are beyond our everyday understanding and so it is not always possible to be confident that someone's beliefs are false.

Just as with voices, some people are not troubled by their unusual beliefs or different understandings of the world and they don't have a negative impact on their lives. We think that you are free to see the world however you like, if it isn't causing you or anyone else any problems! However, other people, such as mental health workers or family members, may say that you 'lack insight', because you don't accept your beliefs and experiences are part of a mental health problem. So, although your beliefs and experiences may not trouble you, they may bring you into conflict with other people and it's important to take this into account when thinking about how to manage them.

If you are troubled by your ideas, or they bring you into conflict with other people then there are two different approaches to managing them, depending on how you answer this question:

Would you rather think that it was all in your mind or would you rather think that it was really happening?

I'd rather think it was all in my mind, so how can I tell if it's really happening?

Unusual beliefs like paranoia can be understood using the same model of distress we described in chapter three. Unusual beliefs are often triggered by things that you notice (e.g.: someone looking at you, something strange in your path, something odd about how you feel). You have thoughts about why it's happening and they influence how you feel and behave, which can in turn have an influence on how you think. For example, if you notice someone looking at you, you might think they are watching you and even planning to harm you, which would naturally make you afraid. Your body would go into 'fight or flight' and you would try and get away as quickly as possible, and you would perhaps try not to go out on your own in future in order to stay safe. When you did go out you'd probably be thinking about the possibility of someone watching you, so you'd be on the look out for it and that would make it more likely that you would notice signs that might mean people were watching you.

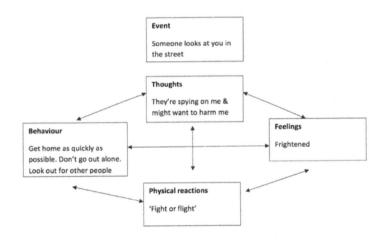

You can try and change any of the different parts that make up your emotional reaction to things you notice. We always think doing something to switch off your 'fight or flight' response, and reduce how scared you feel is a good place to start, as it can help you think more clearly. You can look back at chapter three to remind yourself how to do that. You can also try mindfully noticing that you are having suspicious thoughts and allowing them to pass, as we described in chapter four but if you're finding this difficult you can also try and challenge your thoughts. Many people ask us how to tell if their beliefs are really happening and we think that the best you can do is take a scientific approach.

The scientific method has been developed over the last couple of hundred years as the most reliable way we of have of knowing what is really going on in the world. You start with a hypothesis, a hunch about what is happening and then you look for evidence for that hunch. If the evidence doesn't fit with your hunch, you come up with another one and see if there is more evidence for that. So when you notice something strange happening it can be helpful to think about what evidence you have and whether or not it supports your idea.

Here is an example:

You notice that the cup of tea you are drinking tastes funny and you think that someone might be trying to poison you.

Evidence for	Evidence against
The tea tastes funny You've been feeling tired a lot recently You've noticed people looking at you strangely in the street	You haven't been sick There has been no sign of a break in Tea can taste funny if the water isn't fresh The milk has been in the fridge for a long time and is nearly past its sell by date You haven't done anything that would make people want to hurt you People don't often go around poisoning other people

It can also be helpful to try and think of other explanations for the evidence which supports your idea. You could make a list of the other possible explanations and rate how likely you think they are, then compare this to how likely your original explanation is:

Other explanations for feeling tired	Likelihood (out of 10)
You haven't been sleeping well	7/10
Your medication makes you tired	8/10
You haven't been eating properly	3/10
You are being poisoned	4/10

Weighing up the evidence in this way can help you decide which is the most likely explanation. There is also a scientific principle you can use, called Occum's razor. This states that when there is more than one possible explanation for something, you should accept the simplest explanation. It can be helpful to try and work out just what would need to be in place for your beliefs to be true:

- How many people would need to be involved?
- What kind of technology would they need to have?
- How much would it cost?
- What would be the point of using all these resources to target you?

This can help you see whether your initial explanation is actually feasible and weigh up how likely it is to be the best explanation.

You might not have much evidence for any of your explanations to start off with, so you might need to look for more and sometimes asking someone you trust to help you can be useful. Other people often see situations in very different ways: if you've ever had a family discussion about something that happened a long time ago you'll know that each member of the family remembers it differently, and probably has a different opinion about it. So, it can be helpful to get an outside perspective on the situation and if you're struggling to come up with an alternative explanation, someone else will usually be able to suggest one for you.

As we said in chapter three, its important not to avoid going into situations you are scared of, so that you can learn that you can cope in them, or that nothing bad will happen. This is because going back into the situation will help you find evidence to tell you what is really happening. However, if you go into the situation looking for signs of what you think is happening, you will almost certainly notice things that you can interpret in that way. So, its important to go in with an open mind, or even to deliberately look for evidence that doesn't support your explanation, so that you can make a fair judgement. So, in the example above, you could try and notice how many times you have a cup of tea and it doesn't taste funny.

Understandably, people can find it difficult to think that they might have misunderstood a situation, as it can leave them feeling foolish or that they must be completely crazy. We think that unusual ideas are a reflection of real, distressing things that have happened to us, so we develop them for a good reason. It seems that unusual beliefs can develop out of painful feelings caused by one situation, that get carried over into other situations, where they don't really belong; we'll discuss this more in chapter nine. This means that rather than having to choose between something being real and you being crazy, you can think of yourself as someone who is having an understandable emotional reaction to something.

I'd rather accept that the situation was really happening

As we said, we can't be sure what is really happening (although the methods used above can be a useful guide) and sometimes accepting that the situation is real seems like a better option. Again, it's important to think about the impact this will have on your life overall and your relationships with people who are important to you: How can you balance accepting your experiences with other things that matter or other people's views of the situation?

59

Building on the work by Romme and Escher with people who hear voices, Tamasin Knight did some research with people who have unusual beliefs, asking about ways that they coped with them, rather than trying to challenge or change them. As everyone's beliefs are different, everyone needs to figure out their own personal coping strategies for the situation that worries them but Tamasin identified a number of different kinds of strategies that people use, which could help you think of your own:

- Start by **reading up** on your experiences, as there may be expert knowledge around that you can draw on. For example, there is lots of useful literature around on defending yourself from witchcraft and psychic attack or warding off aliens.
- You can use this information to help you think about how you might be able to **protect yourself**: for example, by wearing special clothing or carrying a charm. You might need to think about how to do this in a way that isn't obvious or doesn't look strange to other people, for example by wearing it under ordinary clothing.
- See if you can find **other people** who have experienced the same thing: there are support groups and internet forums for people who have experienced all kinds of threats and persecution, from alien abduction to the security services. Sharing your concerns with other people and hearing how they cope with them can be very helpful.
- Find ways to build your **self-esteem** and a positive identity: it is much easier not to be bothered by persecution if we feel confident in ourselves. Finding things you are good at and people who value you can help. Some people find it helpful to remember that going through difficult experiences makes them stronger, so that they see themselves as survivors rather

than victims. We encourage people to think about ways in which they might still be able to have a good life, even though they are experiencing threats and challenges.

Tamasin suggests trying to problem solve by asking yourself these questions:
- What do I want or need?
- What is stopping me from getting that (the obstacle)?
- What is the ultimate goal I am trying to achieve?
- How can I get round the obstacle to achieve my goal in a different way?

You can read more in Tamasin's book Beyond Belief, which is available free online from Peter Lehmann Publishing.

Melanie's experience

Many people have unusual beliefs. The more I talk to people the more I realise that humans generally do have unusual thoughts and what can seem like strange beliefs.
My unusual beliefs no longer get in the way of my life. When I was psychotic I acted very weirdly, but most people have been kind and do not hold it against me. There have been times when these beliefs were overwhelming. I have thought the people on the television were talking to me and about me, I thought the world would come to end if I didn't do certain things. Like many people with psychosis I believed I was the chosen one, the new messiah. It gave my life a spiritual meaning and a reason for being in the world. Now I work in mental health, although I'm not saving the world, I do believe I can make a difference. That belief is now not so important to me, or rather it is expressed in a different way.
When I was psychotic I was fastidious and highly emotionally charged about what I would eat and drink and I walked incessantly but only on concrete so I wouldn't harm any insects in the grass. I also lectured people about what

they needed to eat to avoid dying or destroying the planet. My close friend told me afterwards that when I was psychotic I seemed more real and complete to her, because she could see the unedited version. In my real life I do try to help people in my work. I do try to eat healthily. I am kind to animals and a vegetarian. I still try to protect the environment. I do believe in God and in a spiritual dimension and my beliefs now connect me with other people rather than separate me from them.

There is an element of 'normal' or at least an explanation for all my unusual thoughts, they do not seem random and at the time they make perfect sense.

In essence my unusual thoughts are not that unusual. These thoughts just take over my life when I am psychotic and my behaviour causes upset and anxiety to those around me. They become stranger and more chaotic when I am in hospital and feeling despair. The more overwhelmed I become the more I cannot contain my thoughts or let them go; I become obsessive about them and they grow bigger in my mind and take over.

I am still learning to talk and joke about what is on my mind so it does not fester and become poisonous or take over. I think this way of letting go of difficult thoughts can take a lifetime to learn. I am not always successful. But I do find talking helps and having trustworthy, empathic and friendly people around helps no end.

Now I believe for example that the birds I see are giving me meaningful messages, but I can cope with these thoughts and they don't stop me enjoying all the other things I have in my life. Maybe the feelings that these thoughts evoke are more positive and easier to live with. In fact it allows me to enjoy nature more and hopefully see a more spiritual side of life. Some say God Himself is a delusion but it is through this search for meaning that I find sense in the world and I am not harming anybody.

Section for reflection:

What unusual beliefs or understandings of the world do you have? Do these trouble you? Do they bring you into conflict with other people? Would you rather they were all in your mind or that the situation was really happening?

What evidence do you have to support your belief? Can you think of another explanation that has more evidence? How could you test if your belief was true? What else would need to be in place for these things to be really happening?

How does your understanding of the world cause you problems? Can you think of things that could keep you safe? Can you think of ways that you could still get what you want out of life despite this happening?

Chapter 7. Using anti-psychotic medication

Almost everybody who experiences psychosis is offered medication and most people end up taking it, even if they don't really want to. In this chapter we will be discussing anti-psychotic medication, although many people are also prescribed other medications, including anti-depressants, mood stabilisers, sleep aids and medications to help with anxiety. If you want more information about any of these medications, there is a list of resources at the end of this chapter.

How does anti-psychotic medication work?

You may have been told that psychosis is caused by a chemical imbalance in the brain. Your brain is made up of millions of nerve cells, which send messages between each other using chemicals called neurotransmitters. It is widely believed that psychosis occurs when there is too much of a neurotransmitter called dopamine in your brain. So, the anti-psychotic medications work by blocking the part of the brain cells which receive messages, so that the dopamine can't get through. However, there is a lot of uncertainty about the relationship between brain chemistry and psychosis, so it is not possible to say that anti-psychotic medication is treating the cause of the problem. Some people think that medication works by having a general sedating effect, making you feel calm and emotionally detached. Many people do find this effect helpful, as it can help to get overwhelming thoughts and feelings back under control, allowing them to focus or rest: a lot of people find that it helps them just to get some sleep. If you look back at our way of understanding distress in chapter three, you can see how it might help by changing your physical reactions to thinking you are under threat, so it could help you to think more clearly and not get caught up in unhelpful patterns of behaviour.

Weighing up the advantages and disadvantages of taking medication

Unfortunately, the sedating effect often goes beyond just working on troubling thoughts and people taking anti-psychotic medications tend to have a lot of trouble with feeling tired, slowed down, numb and de-motivated. Other common side effects are:

- Weight gain and risk of diabetes
- Tremor or shaking
- Drooling
- Restlessness
- Sexual difficulties

Some people have found ways of coping with these effects. Here is a summary of strategies that a group of people taking anti-psychotics in Australia found helpful in managing tiredness or sedation and weight gain:

Sedation/tiredness

Do's:
• Try to establish normal day/night routines – i.e. up during the day and in bed at night
• Take short naps in the morning (but not in the afternoon)
• Plan your day – arrange tasks when tiredness likely – do the shopping, go for a walk, telephone a friend
• Have a reason for getting up in the morning – have a pet to feed, a job to go to, a hobby, something to do
• Start the day with a shower or splash cold water on face
• Have a cup of coffee to get going or when feeling tired
• Eat an apple for breakfast – apples help to combat tiredness
• Take evening medication about 30 minutes prior to bedtime
• Positive thinking – "I can beat this"

Don'ts:
• Stay in bed late into the morning even if feeling tired
• Take naps in afternoon or prior to bedtime

• Watch TV in bed
• Exercise or eat large meals prior to bedtime
• Drink coffee or tea in the late afternoon or prior to bedtime

Weight gain

Do's:
• Eat smaller meals throughout the day; drink lots of water during day
• Carry an apple or piece of fruit to eat when feeling hungry
• Suck on ice cubes made from juice when hungry
• Build exercise into your daily routine – e.g. go for a walk or do exercise 3–4 times a week
• Be mindful of opportunities to exercise – cycle/walk to places rather than catch transport, use stairs rather than a lift
• Try to avoid boredom – get a hobby, exercise
• Take medications later in the evening – this helps to prevents cravings for food before bedtime
• Learn to cook your own food
• Substitute foods containing high levels of fat and or sugar with low fat/sugar options

Don'ts:
• Eat takeaway foods more than a couple of times a week
• Keep chocolate in the fridge or biscuits in the home
• Give in to weight gain – remain positive

As everyone's brain is unique (reflecting their genetic make-up and their individual life-history), it is not possible to predict what effect any particular medication will have on them. So, we can tell from research what effects a medication is likely to have (because it has that effect on a certain proportion of people who take it), but you can only find out what effect it will have on you by actually taking it. That goes for both the helpful and unhelpful effects: although anti-psychotic medications are widely recommended, and many people do get some benefit from them, there is also evidence that some people do not get much benefit. Because of this, many people wonder whether it is worth taking anti-psychotic medication. As only you can know how the medication affects you, this is something that you have to think through for yourself, although it's also worth asking other people who you trust to help you think it through, as sometimes they can bring a different perspective.

We use the same approach for weighing up the advantages and disadvantages of anti-psychotic medication as we do for other drugs (see chapter three) and again we've filled in some examples based on people we've met:

Pros (benefits) of taking medication	Cons (costs) of taking medication
Helps to make voices quieter Helps me sleep Makes me calmer	Putting on weight Feel tired a lot Feel like 'odd one out'
Pros (benefits) of not taking medication	Cons (costs) of not taking medication
Wouldn't always have to be remembering to take it Feel more motivated Less risk of long term health problems	Harder to cope with stress Psychosis may come back

Can I come off anti-psychotic medication?

In the past, many psychiatrists believed that people would need to take anti-psychotic medication for the rest of their lives. However, this is changing, as there is increasing evidence, from research and people who have shared their experiences, that some people can successfully come off anti-psychotic medications. These people either do not experience their difficulties coming back, or find other ways to manage them. Again, it's important to remember that everyone is different: some people try unsuccessfully to come off medication and we aren't sure about what makes it possible for some people to succeed in coming off and not others.

It does seem that people who have worked on developing other coping strategies may be more likely to be able to reduce or stop their medication. We like the idea of 'personal medicines' developed by Pat Deegan (who we mentioned in chapter two). She describes these as the things that you do to be well, rather than the things that you take, 'the smaller things we do to take care of ourselves and to manage our distress' like:

- Playing with my dog helps me forget my troubles

- Taking care of my daughter gives me a reason to get well

- Reading the bible   each evening calms me and helps me feel strong

There are withdrawal effects of coming off anti-psychotic medications which can make it difficult to come off. This is because our brain cells adjust to the dopamine messages not getting through by becoming more sensitive to dopamine, in an attempt to continue to try and receive the messages. This means that when the medication which is blocking the dopamine is taken away, the receiving cells will be flooded with dopamine and this can trigger psychotic experiences. This effect can happen even when someone has never previously experienced psychosis (so they may have been taking these medications for other reasons) and so is simply an effect of the withdrawal. However, it is often seen as a relapse of the original problem.

In order to prevent this 'rebound psychosis' it is important to reduce the dose of anti-psychotics very gradually. It is recommended that you reduce your medication by ten percent at a time and that if you have been on it for many years that you should do this over the course of at least twelve months. You can find more advice in the section below about where to find information about medication. If you do plan to reduce your medication, you should discuss this with your doctor and mental health workers, as they should support you in thinking through your options and making a plan to help you manage this.

Melanie's experiences

Few people want to take pharmaceutical medication, even for clearly understood physical illnesses. People want to take it even less when it has unpleasant side effects. It is upsetting to withdraw from medication and initially feel wonderful and energetic and then, when chaos descends, the drugs are literally forced into me.

I am now resigned to take the tablets and I think I may have to take them for a long time.

There are two particular side effects that I dislike intensely. The first is weight gain; I gained six stone in six months when I started to swallow the antipsychotics. As a single young woman trying to establish a life for myself the weight gain was horrendous. The rest of my family is naturally slim as I always was in the past, but now I can eat forever and not feel satiated.

The second is sedation. I feel tired a lot of the time and getting up in the morning is a struggle most days. In the past I was always jumping out of bed with the birdsong and needed little rest, this has all changed since taking the tablets.

Another reason I dislike taking the medication is the slick marketing and profiteering of the pharmaceutical companies. Calling them anti-psychotics is basically dishonest because they do not actually get rid of the psychosis, voices etc. It would be more honest to market them as neuroleptics or major tranquilizers, as that is what they do. They put my brain to rest. They stop me feeling and thinking too much but they do not stop the unusual experiences or hallucinations. They make me appear normal because I no longer get so upset by what is going on in my head. I feel calm, rational and able to think more coherently, even if I think paranoid thoughts they no longer bother me.

When I reflect on the benefits of the medication, I have to acknowledge that now my mood is stable, my emotional responses are within the normal range and I can function. I can sleep, eat, work, drive, maintain our home, and look after our cat. I can organise holidays and enjoy the change of scene and adventure. I can keep myself safe and not alienate myself or cause undue stress to others.

It is mainly on the on the wishes of my loved ones that I am so compliant. Each night I am tempted to try to reduce my dose but it is the thought of the upset and anxiety I could cause my husband, my family, my friends, colleagues, (and anyone else) that I carry on taking the 400 mg of Amisulpride each night. There are very important people in my life that need me to be consistent, (the way I am on medication), and these people matter more to me than the intense feelings that I think I am missing out on. When I stop the tablets I have unmanageable experiences, even if I feel better. I am in danger of losing the relationships and connections that I live for.

The last time I was in hospital I was offered (but not forced) to take a mood stabilising medication (Lithium) as well as the antipsychotic, but I declined. I have never had unmanageable problems with high or low moods since.

I feel relieved that I only need to take one type of medication and it helps me live the life I want. I have felt like a failure in the past for not being able to manage without it. I thought this meant I had a weaker personality and I was lacking in self awareness but I am learning the value of accepting myself the way I am and not comparing myself to people who manage without medication. Of course there are millions of people in the UK on long term medication that enables them to get on with their lives.

Where can I get more information to help me make decisions about medication?

Websites
- 'Choice and medication' website: has lots of information about all the different mental health medications and 'handy charts' to help you compare likely side effects:
  www.choiceandmedication.org/devon
- Mind website: has information about all the different mental health medications and a section on coming off medication:
  http://www.mind.org.uk/information-support/drugs-and-treatments/medication/
  http://www.mind.org.uk/information-support/drugs-and-treatments/medication-stopping-or-coming-off/
- 'Coming off' website: has lots of information about all the different mental health medications and advice on how to withdraw from them.
  www.comingoff.com

Book
- Psychiatric Drugs: A Straight talking Guide by Joanna Moncrieff (published by PPCS Books)

Film
- Coming Off Psych Drugs: A Meeting of the Minds by Daniel Mackler (available on You Tube)

Section for reflection:

What are the advantages and disadvantages of your medication for you?

Are there any ways you could manage the side effects better?

What other ways do you have of coping with your difficulties? What are your 'personal medicines'?

Chapter 8. Understanding your experiences: Are they caused by an illness?

In the next three chapters, we will be exploring different ways of making sense of psychosis. The stories of people who have recovered, or learnt to live well, after experiencing psychosis, suggest that is helpful to have a way of understanding it that make sense to you and helps you connect to other people.

There are lots of different ideas about what causes psychosis, but there is no strong evidence that any of them is true, or the only explanation. This means that there is no right way of understanding what has happened to you, so we'll be looking at some of the different ideas and you can think about which work best for you. We take the view that a good explanation is one that helps you get on with your life and do the things you value. We think it's helpful to ask yourself these questions:

- How would I feel if this idea was true?

- Would it make me feel more or less in control?

- Would it make me feel better or worse about myself?

- Would it make me more or less connected to other people?

Isn't psychosis caused by a brain disease?

Many people are told that their experiences are caused by a mental illness. There are debates about exactly what this means, as for some people it simply means that what they are experiencing is very challenging and distressing or prevents them from living the life they want. In this chapter we are using 'mental illness' to refer to the medical (or bio-medical) model of psychosis, which looks for causes in biology and the functioning of the brain. The bio-medical model sees psychosis as the symptoms of a genetic brain disease. People with the genes thought to be linked to this disease will have brains that are abnormal in some way, either the structure of the brain, the brain chemistry or both. There are lots of different ideas about the exact detail of how brain biology leads to psychosis. However, there is only limited evidence that this is broadly the right way of thinking about psychosis, so we encourage people to think about the advantages and disadvantage of this idea. Below are some examples from discussions we've had in the group:

Pros	Cons
• You know what's wrong with you • Doctors will have the answers • It' s easy to explain to other people • It lets you off the hook: it's not your fault	• Stigma: people are scared • You feel as if there's something wrong with you • Feel helpless: there's nothing you can do about it • It lets you off the hook: people have lower expectations, it's an excuse not to do hard things

Some people find it reassuring to think that their experiences are caused by a mental illness but for others it can make them feel as if there's nothing they can do about it, that it's down to doctors to come up with treatments to make you better. We've learnt from the stories of people who've experienced recovery that starting to take control and discovering what you can do to help yourself is important and that doesn't fit that well with the bio-medical model. We'll be looking at some alternative ideas in the next couple of chapters.

Melanie's experiences

For the first few years after I was given the diagnosis 'schizophrenia' I thought that psychosis was an illness. I believed if I listened to the doctors and spent time in hospital I would get better and be fixed. I traipsed from one out patient appointment to the next and tried nearly every type of medication until my expectation of a cure slowly died and gave way to a life of self management and acceptance.

I have sought answers from every kind of expert until I realised and learnt that I was the expert on my experiences and no one would know me better than I know myself.

Now I see psychosis as being on the extreme end of the sensitivity spectrum, with a vulnerability to the demands of relationships, work, life, and society. It can be viewed as a gift, a mode of slipping into another world that is inaccessible to many. Sometimes I feel isolated and lonely in my own mind, but when I slip into a psychotic world I am escaping this. I also see it as a spiritual experience, an emergence of another realm.

When I realised there is no quick fix for my condition I needed to find my own way through, for me this has been finding meaning and purpose in my experiences and using it to help others. Empathy and helping others goes a long way and is a great way to help yourself too.

Acute psychosis may be a result of lacking whatever it takes to cope in the world, but it has also given me magical, exhilarating experiences in this 'other' life. For example I have 'seen' a star being created and I have felt as big as the entire universe and as small as an embryo. These experiences can feel amazing, and take my breath away.

I no longer believe I am ill and I do not seek a cure for my feelings or unusual experiences. I do not subscribe to the medical model or think I am ill when I have experienced things that don't fit into the schema that society wants or needs to operate in.

Society needs a certain amount of order and conformity to function, and balancing boundaries and freedoms can have personal rewards too. Labelling and controlling people with psychosis enables others to feel normal and well in comparison.

Now I feel as well as anybody else and I view my individual differences as a positive addition to my life. The other/psychotic dimension that I live with provides richness and originality to my thoughts and character that I would not want to be without.

Section for reflection:

Have you been told that your experiences are caused by an illness? How does this make you feel about yourself and your life?

What are the advantages and disadvantages for you of the biomedical model?

Chapter 9. Understanding your experiences: the impact of life events

Some people think that rather than being an illness which you inherit, psychosis is a reaction to the things that happen to you in your life. They think that psychosis is a 'sane response to living in a crazy world'. Again, there is no proof that this idea is definitely true but most people do believe that stress can trigger psychotic experiences.

The stress-vulnerability model

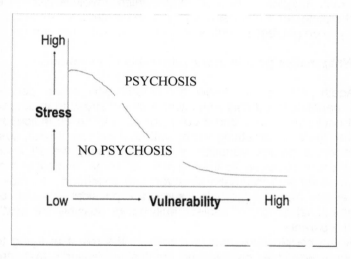

This diagram shows that it is possible for anyone to experience psychosis if they are put under enough stress. However, some people are more vulnerable than others, meaning that it takes lower levels of stress to trigger psychotic experiences in them.

Most people are able to identify that they went through a period of stress at the times their difficulties started. People who hear voices have described these life events happening to them before the experience started:

- Bereavement
- Falling in love

- Serious illness of someone close
- Divorce / relationship breakdown
- Failing at school / college
- Violence between parents
- Pregnancy / birth in family

You might notice that some of these life events are usually associated with happy feelings and its important to remember that happy events can be as stressful as sad or upsetting events. Research into the impact of stress on health suggests that anything which involves your life changing, for the better or worse, can be stressful, especially if you do not feel in control or able to deal with that change.

What makes people more vulnerable to psychosis?

Again, we do not know for certain why some people experience psychosis with lower levels of stress than others. It could be genetic and it does not have to be an indication that there is something wrong with that person: it could just reflect a natural variation, in the same way we all have different physical abilities. There is some evidence that upsetting and traumatic life events in childhood can make people more vulnerable, such as physical, sexual or emotional abuse, or neglect, bullying, or possibly the death of a parent.

Some people think that psychosis is the result of trying to cope with the painful and confusing feelings that are associated with traumatic events, by blocking them out. When we are experiencing an upsetting event, its often not safe for us to show feelings like fear or anger, so we tend to put them to one side. If we don't get the chance to deal with those feelings later, they can come back in the form of psychosis. So, one way to understand the experience of hearing voices is that the voices represent the feelings that someone has put away and maybe tried to forget about. Another idea is that feelings we've had in upsetting situations get separated off from our memory of what actually happened, and then the feeling can come back on its own, without us knowing why we're having it. This could be a feeling in our body or an emotional state, like feeling like somebody is trying to hurt you. Because this is very confusing, we then try and come up with an explanation for why we are feeling this way and sometimes those explanations can be very unusual, because it is hard to face the real reasons we have the feelings. So, it can be helpful to try and see if there are metaphorical or emotional connections between psychotic experiences and events that have happened in your life. So, if your experiences leave you feeling very vulnerable, you could think about times in your life when you might have felt vulnerable.

For these reasons, it can be helpful to try and understand your feelings better and find ways of expressing them. Its often helpful to find someone you trust to talk through your life events and feelings about them, but if this is too difficult writing them down, in a journal or expressing them creatively can also be helpful.

The effect of life events on beliefs about ourselves and others

Psychologists think that another way that life events can contribute to psychosis is through their impact on our beliefs about ourselves and others. To understand this, think for a moment about how experiences like being bullied or emotionally abused, through being criticised and put down, might make someone feel:

- About themselves
- About other people

Usually what people end up feeling is worthless and small, maybe even that they deserve to be treated badly. They might also learn that other people can't be trusted and are likely to hurt them.

So, now think about what it would mean if the voices you hear were telling the truth about you, or if the unusual beliefs you have really were true:

- About yourself
- About other people

You might find this is very similar, that the voices seem to think you are small and worthless and deserve to be treated badly and that other people want to hurt you.

Psychologists believe that when someone is treated badly, they develop beliefs about themselves that they are no good and that people will always treat them badly. This means that they are much more likely to interpret things that happen to them as signs that these beliefs are true. If you look back at the way of understanding emotions we described in chapter three, you will see that our interpretations are important in how we feel about and react to events, including hearing voices. Our interpretations and thought processes are driven by our 'core beliefs', so if we've grown up feeling under threat and that we're no good, we'll be quick to see everything that happens to us in that way.

Sometimes psychosis can actually to lead to people feeling very positive about themselves, that they are special or particularly good, rather than the opposite. It's a strange idea but psychologists think that this can be a way of coping with, or protecting yourself against, feeling like you are bad, trying to keep these painful feelings as far outside your mind as possible. Feeling really good about yourself can bring its own problems, because it can mean you take big risks or do things that upset other people because you care less about what they think.

Working on problematic beliefs about yourself and others

As core beliefs can fuel psychosis, it can be helpful to try and change them. It can be helpful to understand the difference between *facts* and *opinions:*

- *Facts*: are supported by evidence and can be measured so that people cannot disagree about them (so how much you weigh is a fact)
- *Opinions*: are based on personal views and can be argued (so thinking you should lose weight is an opinion)

Although our core beliefs can feel like they are simply true, they are opinions, not facts and so we can change them. Here are some useful strategies:

- Core beliefs are usually 'all or nothing', eg: ' I'm completely useless', 'no-one cares about me'. As the world isn't black and white like this, it can be quite straightforward to find a counter-example, of something useful you did or something caring someone has done. This can help you re-evaluate your beliefs.

- Try and think about a time that you felt good about yourself, or that people did something nice, even if it was just for a few seconds. How did that make you feel about yourself and other people? Once you've done that, can you think of other times you felt that way?

- Make a list of your strengths: things you're good at, things people compliment you on, things you're proud of.

- Ask other people what they like or admire about you.

- Try writing down all these other possible beliefs about yourself, so that when your voices or unusual ideas get you feeling that you're no good or people will always hurt you, you can remind yourself.

The aim here isn't to get you thinking that you're completely brilliant and the world is a lovely place: like we said that can be unhelpful too and is also not a realistic representation of reality. These exercises are to try and help you find a balanced perspective. We think that the most helpful way of seeing ourselves and other people is to accept that we all have strengths and weaknesses. Sometimes bad things happen, and this can make us feel bad but there are good things, and good people in life too.

Melanie's experiences

There is not any one reason why I developed psychosis. There are too many possible explanations. With the benefit of hindsight, it was like the perfect storm and my life couldn't really have gone any other way.

My Aunty had psychosis for years until she died and this may have made my own experience genetically more likely. My father has also got a mental health problem although he has never been psychotic.

At four years of age I experienced a trauma that I couldn't speak to anyone about and I shut it away in the back of my mind as if it was forgotten. I believe this was a big factor in my later psychosis.

I have had several accidental bangs to the head that rendered me unconscious. Head injuries are sometimes though to affect mental health.

My family immigrated to the UK from Canada when I was nine years old, and moving overseas can make mental health vulnerabilities more likely.

Immediately after moving to England my parents had a very acrimonious divorce and family breakdown is another possible factor.

As a teenager I had a difficult relationship with a man who was abusive and again I felt I had no one I could confide in. It also put me off having relationships for a very long time. I think this emotional isolation was another trigger for my psychosis.

I started to smoke cannabis with my friends but I was the only one who became psychotic. It possibly made me more paranoid and my mental health more vulnerable.

While the psychosis was taking hold of my mind I was living, working and studying away from home in relative poverty. I lived in an inner city environment with all the stress, noise, crime and pollution that came with it. Mental health problems are more prevalent in inner cities.

The beginning of my first psychotic episode at university when I was nineteen years old felt much like a trauma flashback and I was reminded by all my hallucinating senses as if I was four year old again. It felt like the experience was coming back to me in pieces of repressed memory and scared and confused feelings. I see this as my unconscious mind spilling over, as trauma cannot remain shut away forever.

All these factors will have made me more susceptible to developing psychosis. In summary I believe it was caused by cumulative stress and vulnerability. By working through my personal history to this point and making sense of why psychosis arose, it has given me clues as to what is contributing to my wellness now.

I cannot go back and change anything. All I can do is make the most of it and hope that any hardships in the past have given me strength and resilience to live my life now. And I appreciate all the positive lessons I have learnt about how to stay as mentally well as possible.

Section for reflection:

Are you aware of any stressful events that may have triggered your experience of psychosis?

Can you think of any difficult events in your past that may have contributed to your psychosis? How might you be able to work through your feelings about this, through talking to someone, writing them down or expressing them creatively?

What are your core beliefs about yourself and other people? If you have any negative core beliefs, can you think of some more positive alternative beliefs?

Chapter 10. Understanding your experiences: spiritual frameworks

As we said in chapter six, for some people unusual experiences and beliefs are simply real events, even though they may be beyond everyday or scientific understanding. Many cultures and religions around the world have other ways of understanding experiences like voices and visions and are made up of belief systems that do not fit with modern Western thought. As we don't think there is a right way to view the world, we think that these ideas can be helpful to people in making sense of their experiences, and finding a way forward from them. As with other ways of making sense of your experience, the important thing is whether it makes sense to you and connects you to other people.

Spirituality can also be an important part of recovery, however you understand your unusual experiences. Many people think that spirituality means belonging to a particular religion and if they don't, they don't think it applies to them. Sometimes people have had bad experiences with religion and so they prefer to avoid it. However, spirituality has a wider meaning and can be an important part of wellbeing for many people. Some people say that their experience of psychosis made them much more aware of their spiritual needs and the importance of finding ways to express their spirituality. There is no agreed definition of spirituality but it is generally about:

- The values, beliefs and ideas that give your life meaning and purpose
- A sense of belonging and connectedness
- Going beyond the individual and the material world
- A greater being or force than humanity or yourself

Having these experiences and ideas can help people to cope with mental health difficulties, by helping them feel that they are not alone, that their troubles are part of a bigger picture, or giving them another focus, outside of themselves and their problems. Things that people do to develop or express their spiritual side include:

- Being in nature
- Praying or dedicating something they do to a higher power
- Meditating
- Creative and expressive activities, like painting or dancing
- Appreciating beauty for example in art or music
- Physical movement: yoga, Tai Chi or even just running

Psychosis could be a breakthrough not a breakdown

Some people think that unusual experiences can be the result of a spiritual crisis, when someone's mind becomes open to the possibility of a new level of awareness and a greater connection to a spiritual realm. The idea that some experiences of psychosis could be a form of 'spiritual emergency' led to the formation of the Spiritual Emergence Network in the USA and more recently the Spiritual Crisis Network in the UK. These organisations offer support to people going through this experience, so that they can learn and grow from them.

There are lots of different belief systems describing the nature of the spiritual realm, which also offer guidance on how to manage connection with it. The major religions offer explanations for unusual experiences, such as demon possession in Christianity and invisible spirits called jinn in Islam. If you already belong to a religion or feel drawn to the teachings of a particular faith, you could contact your local faith leader to ask for their advice on what you are experiencing. They may be able to help you understand the teachings of that faith and how they apply to you. They may also be able to offer prayers, forgiveness or perform ceremonies related to what you are experiencing.

There are some other, less well known approaches that some people we know have found useful:

Shamanism

In traditional cultures, shamans alter their states of mind in order to enter into the spirit realm and seek advice and healing, often from animal spirit guides. Shamans usually enter a trance state through a ritual and so have a controlled way of accessing and leaving the spirit world. Shamanic training can also help people to learn how to channel and interpret their contacts with spirits, so that they do not become overwhelming or destructive.

Spiritualism

Spiritualism is a more modern belief system, linked to Christianity. Spiritualists believe that some people, called mediums, have the ability to communicate telepathically with the spirits of dead people. Anyone can develop this gift but there are ways of tuning it and spiritualist churches and groups offer support and training. As well as helpful and positive spirits (e.g.: angels and people who were positive while they were alive) there are also negative spirits (e.g. demons and people who did bad things while they were alive), which tend to be drawn to people who are vulnerable, often because they have suffered trauma. It is thought that this fragments the soul and causes a hole in someone's aura, allowing the negative spirit access and that taking drugs like cannabis can have this effect too. There are strategies for defending yourself against such negative influences, often called psychic self-defence and spiritualist churches and practitioners can offer support, guidance and healing. There is also an understanding that just as living people can be made negative by not having their needs met, spirits can too, so this may involve healing the negative spirits as much as yourself.

There are other belief systems that are relevant to unusual experiences and which some people find helpful in making sense of what is happening to them, such as Kundilini awakening, reincarnation and alien encounters and the general advice below applies to them too. You may need to explore a few different belief systems in order to find one that works for you. As with the other ideas for making sense of your experiences, we'd encourage you to weigh up the advantages and disadvantages of spiritual beliefs too. Here's an example of a discussion from our group:

Pros	Cons
• It means you're special rather than ill • It means that you can get some new insight from your experience • It means you can move forward to a better life • You can find other people who understand and accept your experiences	• People who don't share these beliefs find them strange and frightening • You have to seek out other people with the same ideas • You have to learn and practice new strategies rather than rely on medication

What helps to manage difficult spiritual experiences?

Although there are lots of different beliefs about the nature of spiritual experiences there are some useful general ideas for making them more manageable:

- **Find out more about it**: you can look up the different belief systems we've mentioned on the internet and in the library to see if they fit with what you're experiencing
- **Talk to an expert**: this could be a leader within a church or faith community, who could provide training in a particular practice or carry out a helpful ceremony or ritual. You could also look for a therapist who specialises in transpersonal psychology, which combines modern psychology and spiritual understandings and aims to help people manage spiritual experiences.

- **Join with people who share the same belief:** they will offer support and understanding as well as advice and guidance. Also, be careful who you share your ideas with, in case they find them hard to accept.
- **Staying grounded:** keeping up your connection with the everyday world, through being aware of your surroundings and having a healthy routine are important to prevent yourself being overwhelmed
- **Creating positive energy:** this could be through the use of affirmation and positive statements about yourself. You may also need to re-visit painful past experiences which are making you vulnerable and deal with your feelings about them: talking to someone (possibly in therapy) or writing a journal can help. You can also ask positive spiritual beings to help you in protecting yourself against negative ones.
- **Creating a psychic boundary around yourself:** You can visualise yourself surrounded with white light, surround yourself mentally with a blue bubble, or imagine yourself surrounded by mirrors, which bounce negativity away from you. You can also use salt to absorb and remove negative energy, by dissolving it in water and leaving it around your home or bathing in it.

Melanie's experiences

Some say the difference between religion and spirituality is that 'Religion is for people who don't want to go to hell and spirituality is for people who have already been there' or that 'Spirituality is a personal relationship with the Divine'.

I have always believed in God but now in a more spiritual sense than a religious belief. I do not go to church or read the Bible but my faith is essential to me. I talk to God frequently and believe that He communicates with me too.

I think that my own track up the mountain to God or the divine is unorthodox but it is still a path and I believe that anyone with faith is trying to get to the top of the same mountain we just have different ways of getting there.

When I think of the problems I have had in life including psychosis I think that God gave me these difficulties because I could cope with them. However tough life is, I think if we all put our problems on the table and we could see what everyone else was coping with, we would choose our own problems to pick up again and keep. They are already familiar to us and we are already coping. And if we really knew what problems that other people have we may count ourselves fortunate.

Even terrible grief can have consolations and we can learn and grow through life's difficulties. My spiritual faith makes problems seem more purposeful, as I can learn from them and support and empathise with others.

Search for spiritual meaning gives my emotional life depth and intensity. It has become apparent to me that life is more mysterious and more interesting since having psychosis and I see my reality as a personal subjective experience. When I was acutely psychotic I felt everything was significant, now I still believe this but in a calmer and more socially acceptable way by believing in my intuition and spiritual evolution.

In Deepak Chopra's writings on spiritual success he says, 'Everyone has a purpose in life...a unique gift or special talent to give to others'. I see psychosis as my gift, with which I can empathise and help people.

My faith has been with me through all my psychotic episodes and remains through all the time I am in recovery. My faith is a consistent theme in my life and ultimately gives me hope.

Helpful sources of information

Your local NHS mental health service may have a chaplaincy service, who can support to make contact with local faith leaders with an understanding of mental health.

Spiritual Strategies for Mental Health, published by Speak up Somerset. Available from wwww.artofrecovery.com
http://www.spiritualcrisisnetwork.org.uk/

Accepting Voices by Marius Romme and Sandra Escher. Published by Mind.

Psychic Self-Defence by Dion Fortune. Published by Red Wheel / Weiser

Handbook for the Urban Warrior by The Barefoot Doctor. Published by Piatkus Books.

Section for reflection:

What spiritual ideas and experiences do you have? What gives your life meaning and purpose and makes you feel connected to something bigger than yourself?

How do you express your spirituality? Do you make enough time for spirituality in your life?

Do you think that there could be anything helpful and supportive for you from 'spiritual' connections?

Could your experience of psychosis be a breakthrough rather than a breakdown? What are the systems of belief that are relevant to your experience? Do you need to find out more about them or connect with people who practise them?

Try some of the strategies for helping yourself feel spiritually safer and more in control: do they make a difference?

Chapter 11. Being prepared for setbacks and looking after yourself

When people have managed to move forward from the worst of their difficulties they are often reluctant to think about the possibility that they could come back. It may seem contradictory but being prepared for your difficulties coming back could actually prevent it from happening or reduce the impact should it occur. As psychosis is triggered by stress, and it's almost impossible to avoid stressful situations in life, it's quite likely that things could get worse for you again. If you are prepared for this, you can notice that it's happening and do something early on to prevent your difficulties from getting completely out of control. Even if you don't manage to do this, many people find that making a plan for what they want to happen when things get out of control helps to make the crisis situation feel more manageable and improve more quickly. It can also help the people who may need to step in and take over to know what you would like to happen, so they can respect your choices.

Setbacks can be a vicious cycle

Research has found that there is usually a gradual process of difficulties starting to come back, over a period of about two weeks. At times of stress, people usually have small changes in their thoughts and feelings, which can then build up into more overwhelming experiences. We think that part of this process is people noticing the small changes and worry about things going wrong again, which starts up the pattern of thoughts, feelings and behaviours we described in chapters five and six.

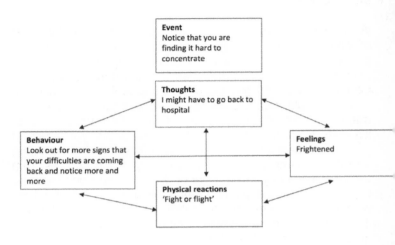

Having a plan for how to manage difficult times can help you to feel less worried about them and so you are less likely to get caught up in this cycle.

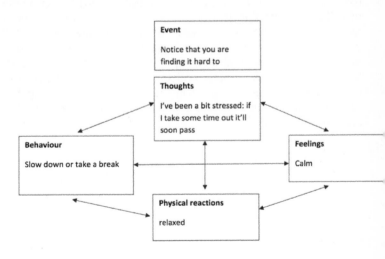

Early warning signs and 'relapse signatures'

The small changes that people have noticed are known as 'early warning signs' and we think that everyone has their own unique pattern of changes, known as a 'relapse signature'. In the box below is a list of common early warning signs that people can have. Think back to the last time you experienced your difficulties getting worse and try and pick out if you noticed any of these changes in the few weeks leading up to that. You might like to ask someone who knows you well what they noticed too, as we don't always notices these changes in ourselves.

Once you have picked out which you experience, think about the order they happened in: did some of the happen earlier and then build up into others? Try and separate them out into early and later stages. Some people find it helpful to make a list of their early warning signs and check how often they are having them. You could do this using the diary format below, recording either if the sign is present or how strong it is on a scale of 0-10. As having some early warning signs doesn't necessarily mean your difficulties are coming back, it is quite likely that you will notice some from time to time. Keeping a record means that you will notice if they are getting any worse.

Thoughts & sensations	Feelings	Behaviours
• Thoughts are racing • Thinking you have special powers • Thinking that other people can read your mind • Thinking that you can read other people's minds • Receiving personal messages from the TV or radio • Having difficulty making decisions • Preoccupied about one or two things • Having difficulty concentrating • Thinking people are talking about you • Senses seem sharper • Experiencing strange sensations • Seeing visions or things other people cannot see • Thinking that a part of you has changed shape • Having more nightmares • Hearing voices • Thinking you might be someone else • Thinking people are against you • Thinking bizarre things • Thinking your thoughts are controlled	• Feeling sad or low • Feeling confused or puzzled • Feeling helpless or useless • Feeling afraid of going crazy • Feeling strong or powerful • Feeling like you're being watched • Feeling increasingly religious • Feeling anxious or restless • Feeling isolated • Feeling tired or lacking energy • Feeling unable to cope with everyday tasks • Feeling like you cannot trust other people • Feeling like you do not need sleep • Feeling guilty • Feeling irritable • Feeling forgetful or far away • Feeling like you are being punished • Feeling in another world	• Not seeing people • Behaving aggressively • Unable to sit down for long • Not eating • Talking or smiling to yourself • Movements are slow • Acting suspiciously as if being watched • Refusing to do simple requests • Behaving like a child • Neglecting your appearance • Not leaving the house • Speech comes out jumbled and filled with odd words • Difficulty in sleeping • Smoking more • Drinking more • Behaving oddly for no reason • Acting like you are someone else • Spending time alone

Sign	M	Tu	W	Th	Fr	Sa	Su

Knowing your triggers

Early warning signs will often start happening because you are in a stressful situation that triggers them off. So, it's helpful to recognise when these situations are happening and then you can think about how to cope with them successfully. Not everyone realises when they are under stress, so to help you think about what might be stressful situations for you, look at the list in the box below. This list is based on some old research into the link between life events and health but we have updated it to make it more relevant. Remember that events associated with positive emotions can be just as stressful as unhappy events: stress is usually caused by feeling out of control and can be part of any loss or change. It can be particularly important to be aware of the impact of events that feel positive because if you're feeling good, you're less likely to be thinking about whether you need to taking more care of yourself.

Death of a partner, close family member or friend
Starting or ending a relationship
Family arguments or family breakdown or spending more or less time with your family
Being injured or ill or someone else in the family being unwell
Getting married or moving in with someone
Getting in trouble at work or losing your job
Leaving your job or retiring, or your partner leaves work or retires
Starting a new job or changes in your current job
Pregnancy or someone else in the family having a baby
Children leaving home
Financial difficulties or having to borrow money
Starting or finishing school, college or other education or changing schools
An outstanding personal achievement
Moving house
Change in habits like sleeping, eating or others
Change in social activities

Although this list suggests that some events are stressful for everyone, different events can be stressful for different people, because of the meanings and associations they have for that person. Usually events that are stressful for us tap into the kind of core beliefs we discussed in chapter nine. So, if you have a belief that you are no good and then someone criticises you or puts you down, that could set off some difficult thoughts and feelings.

Making a plan

There are a few different approaches to making a plan to prevent your difficulties coming back, or keeping some control if they do, known as 'relapse prevention', 'recovery' or 'crisis' plans. In our group, we talk about Wellness

Recovery Action Plans (WRAPs). We like this approach because it was developed by someone who had mental health problems herself and who wanted to learn how to manage her difficulties better rather than relying on medication. (You can learn more about Mary Ellen Copeland on her website, see below). It also encourages people to work on being at their best, not just preventing the worst from happening. We'll look more at improving your wellbeing in chapter twelve.)

The Wellness Recovery Action Plan includes:

- **A wellness toolbox:** make a list of everything you do that makes you feel better. Some examples are: listening to music, patting my dog, going for a walk. You could include some of the ideas from chapter 4 or your personal medicines from chapter 8.

- **A daily maintenance plan:** make a list of things you need to do every day in order to be at your best. Examples are getting 8 hours sleep, eating a healthy meal or being in touch with a friend. You could also include things to do less frequently and things to avoid.

- **Triggers:** make a list of your triggers or situations that might set off difficult thoughts and feelings. Make a list of ways you could avoid them and strategies you could use to cope if they come up. An example of a trigger is being criticised, and you might try and avoid people if you know they often put you down, or if it happens you could contact a friend for reassurance.

- **Early warning signs:** make a list of the first, small changes you might notice that things are getting more difficult and then think about how you might cope with them. An example might be that you are not sleeping well and you could cope by doing some relaxation exercises before bed.

- **When things are breaking down:** make a list of the later, bigger changes you would notice if your difficulties were starting to come back and then think of some strategies you could use to cope with them. An example might be that you begin having suspicious thought and you might want to take some extra medication and look for evidence that your thoughts are not true.

- **Crisis plan or advance directive:** Think about what the signs would be that you have lost control and you need someone else to step in and take care of you or make decisions for you. Make a list of who you would like to support you, what you'd like them to do, anyone you don't want involved, medications and treatments you do and don't want, places you'd like to stay and signs that you are ready to take your life back over.
- **Post-crisis plan:** Think about what help and support you'd need to get back in your feet after a crisis. Also, think about what you might need to do to put right any problems that the crisis might have caused, such as in relationships or at work. Think about what you can learn from the crisis: what worked well, what did not work well and how might you change your WRAP to prevent a similar crisis in future

You can find lots of templates and advice on completing a WRAP online, just by putting Wellness Recovery Action Plan into your search engine. You might like to start by visiting the official WRAP website, where you can also read other people's stories and see examples of their plans and tools: www.mentalhealthrecovery.com

When you complete a plan, its very important that you share it with the people who you want to support you if things get difficult: if they don't know about the plan, they can't use it. If you want or need someone to do something for you as part of your plan it is important to discuss this with them so your plan becomes a record of that agreement rather than a hope for what you'd like to happen.

A WRAP plan is best developed when you are well enough to give it time and energy and can reflect clearly on your experience. People can find it helpful to read their plans frequently, Mary Ellen suggests taking 20 minutes a day to remind yourself of what you have decided you need to do to stay well and the actions you wish to take if things change. A plan is also something that needs to grow and change with you and as your life changes. If you do go through another difficult time, you might learn something new and valuable from it and want to add this to your plan. Although setbacks are difficult, they are also an opportunity to learn, about ourselves and what we need in order to be the best we can be. Gradually you will be able to make a self help manual which you have written yourself on the basis of what, in your experience, works best for you. It can support you in becoming skilful, confident and increasingly resilient as you successfully learn how best to look after yourself and enable others to know what you value and need.

Melanie's experience

Being in recovery has taught me how to live with fluctuating mental health and that I may be vulnerable to setbacks. I wrote a Wellness Recovery Action Plan with someone who also lives with mental health problems; we discussed each section carefully and shared ideas. My plan has evolved, I now know it by heart, and it has been invaluable.

I stay as well as I can by using the Daily Maintenance part of my WRAP plan. It may be small simple things like having a shower, going for a walk, staying in touch with people, taking the tablets, going to bed at a reasonable time, avoiding alcohol and saying 'no' to demands that will put me under too much pressure. There are also things that I remember to do less often than every day like go swimming, go out with friends, go on holiday and get a break from work and from household responsibilities.

Of course it is not possible to avoid stress altogether and things that trigger me are too many demands on my time, and energy, combined with a lack of space to gather my thoughts and spend time pottering around and keeping up with necessary chores.

The first signs that I notice that I am going downhill is that I frown a lot, become argumentative, I find it impossible to sleep properly and I lose my appetite. I start smoking again and look for problems to ruminate on. If I have reduced the medication my family will become anxious and nag me to take the full dose. They warn me I may end up in hospital and they are at the end of their tether with me. All this conflict causes anxiety, we have arguments and they are not satisfied until I relent and take the full dose again. Then they seem satisfied, which makes me relax and feel better.

Over the years I have learnt that the medication is very important to maintain my relationships and my life on an even keel. A few times I have persisted and come off the tablets altogether. I insisted I did not need anyone to tell me what to do. I rebelled and argued with people who I felt wanted me to conform. On my last recurrence of acute psychosis I had left my husband, moved out of my home, gone on long term sick leave from work, overwhelmed my family and friends until eventually I had gone so far that there was no way back. I escaped into my own mind where life was bearable but no one could reach me.

This was when I really needed my Crisis Plan. I needed the staff in hospital to read it and recognise I wasn't always struggling with psychosis, and to see me as a whole person. I had written about what treatment I wanted, and what I could not accept. It helped the staff to see beyond the psychosis and see me as someone who had a full life, and insight into managing my situation. They were able to hold hope for me.

When I am well I am generally positive, upbeat and sociable. I get on well with people and I enjoy life. This is how I recognise myself and give my husband and others space to relax and know that they don't have to worry about me. I also don't need to worry about myself, as I have practical and proven ways of managing my life and my recovery.

Section for reflection:

Do you think you can learn from your experience and use that information to make a plan for what you can do to stay well and take action when things change?

Think back to the last time that things were difficult for you: what small changes did you notice in how you were thinking and feeling?

What do you think your triggers are? How could you avoid them or cope with them better?

What would you like to happen if you lose control and need someone else to take over for a while?

Chapter 12. Living well and moving forward

In chapter three we talked about how recovery is more than just getting your difficult and distressing experiences under control, it's also about living well, whatever that means to you. In chapter eleven, we described how you can use a Wellness Recovery Action Plan to help you be at your best, by developing a wellness toolbox, with ideas about things you can to do help yourself feel better and a daily maintenance plan, to make sure you do those things regularly. There are some areas that people find it particularly helpful to work on to improve their wellbeing.

The five ways to wellbeing

You might know that you are supposed to eat five portions of fruit and vegetables a day in order to be physically healthy. But did you know that there are five types of activity that you should do every day in order to look after your mental health? The government did a large research project to find out what kind of really activities helped people to be mentally healthy. They found that you've a good chance of staying well if you :

Connect with the people around you: your family, friends, colleagues and neighbours. You could take time out to ask how they are or get in touch if you've not heard from them for a while.

keep Learning: you could try something new or pick up and old interest. You could go on a course, learn a new skill like cooking or even just listen to the news or learn a new word.

be Active: most people now believe that exercise is good for mental health as well as physical health. It's important to find something you enjoy and which suits your level of fitness: it could just be going for a walk or taking the stairs but it could be cycling, swimming, dancing or aerobics.

take Notice: this is similar in some ways to mindfulness. It's about paying attention to the world around you, especially things that are beautiful or interesting and take you outside of yourself. It can also help you be aware of what really matters to you and so make the most of your life. You could try noticing something different on a journey you make every day or really paying attention to the food you are eating and how it tastes or focus on other senses such as hearing or smell.

Give: making other people happy can make you happier too. It doesn't have to be a big thing, like doing voluntary work, it could be something small like a random act of kindness or just smiling at people or saying 'thank you'.

You might notice that the capital letters of the five activities spell the word 'CLANG' which can be helpful way of remembering what they are. If you have a smart phone, there is also a free app available, which you can use to remind yourself what to do each day.

Moving forward

There are many similarities between the five ways to wellbeing and the things that support recovery we talked about in chapter three: feeling connected to others, having hope for a better life, having a positive sense of identity, finding meaning in your experiences and your life and feeling in control of your mental health and your life. For many people, opportunities to do the things that support recovery and wellbeing come through going back into work or education or joining a group or team. People who have come to our group have found it particularly helpful to spend time with other people who have experienced the same difficulties as them, as it makes them feel understood and accepted. They've also found having the opportunity to learn more about their difficulties helps them feel more positive and sometimes it just gives them a reason to get out of the house and a structure to the week. The people who have come back after finishing one group to help us run the next one have also felt really good that they can use their experiences to support other people.

You could try and find similar opportunities in your area:

- **Hearing voices groups** are a place where people with unusual experiences can come together and talk about their experiences safely and confidentially. You can see if there is a group near you at: http://www.hearing-voices.org/hearing-voices-groups/

- Hearing voices groups are just one kind of **peer support groups**. Peer support means people who have had similar experiences offering each other help and understanding and it is thought that both giving and receiving support can be helpful to recovery. You can find out about peer support groups in your area at: http://www.mind.org.uk/information-support/guides-to-support-and-services/peer-support/about-peer-support/

- **Recovery colleges** provide courses about mental health and recovery, run by people with personal experience of mental health difficulties working together with mental health workers. They are provided within mental health services and often offer courses on peer support as well as other aspects of recovery. You can search for recovery colleges in your area online.

- **Volunteering with local mental health services**, either in the NHS or with charities like Rethink or Mind. Many of these organisations now see having personal experience of mental health difficulties as a qualification to work for them and some offer peer support worker roles, which are intended to give people a chance to use their personal experience to help others. You may find that these are also available as paid jobs.

- **User involvement**: your local mental health services should have a way of finding out what people using the services think and there may be opportunities for them to get involved in attending meetings, delivering training, sitting on interview panels or carrying out research. You can find out more about what opportunities are available in your area through contacting the Patient Advice and Liaison Service (PALS) at your local NHS mental health service or through finding your local Healthwatch at www.healthwatch.co.uk

Of course, you don't have to do something related to mental health; many people prefer to find work, courses or social groups that have nothing to do with mental health. But, it can be a good way of making something positive out of your experiences and it can sometimes feel easier to start out by doing something where other people understand the difficulties you've had and value your experience.

Overcoming stigma and self-stigma

After experiencing psychosis, many people can find it difficult to rebuild their lives by getting into work, education or social groups because of the stigma associated with psychosis. Stigma is made up of three elements

- **Stereotypes**: these are myths about what people with psychosis are like. Common myths are that people with psychosis are somehow fundamentally different from other people, that they are dangerous or unpredictable, that they cannot live independently or work and they need to be in hospital.
- **Prejudice:** people believe that the myths about psychosis are true
- **Discrimination:** people with psychosis are treated differently because other people believe the myths. So, they may be turned down for jobs or college courses just because they have had psychosis.

Unfortunately people who have psychosis themselves often also believe that the myths about psychosis are true: this is called self-stigma. It means that you have negative views and low expectations of yourself because you have had psychosis. This can lead to something called the 'why try?' effect, when people give up on themselves, which then reinforces their negative views about themselves.

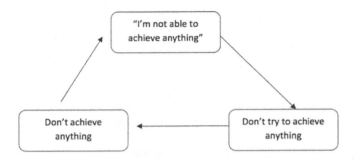

We hope that from this book you have found out that anyone can experience psychosis and they can recover, getting in control of their experiences, going on to live in the same way as many other people, having their own homes, working, getting married and having families. Despite the stories that sometimes appear in newspapers and on TV, people with psychosis are no more dangerous than anyone else and in fact are more likely to be victims of crime, or hurt themselves, than to hurt other people.

You can tackle self stigma by:

- **Building up your self-esteem**: look back at the suggestions in chapter nine for changing your view of yourself.
- **Setting yourself realistic goals** and then celebrate your achievements: managing to do something small will help build your confidence and you can gradually work towards bigger goals. It can help to start with setting a goal that is something you've already done (like making a to-do list where the first item is to make the list!).
- **Practice self-acceptance**: this is where mindfulness can be helpful again, as it encourages you to notice things about yourself without judging them. Try being understanding and forgiving towards yourself, reflecting on the obstacles you've had to face or the good reasons why things have been harder for you. It can be helpful to think how a sympathetic friend or outsider would see your

situation, and think about the things they might say to you. We find the phrase 'you're doing the best you can with what you've got' helpful. It can also be helpful to remember that everyone has a dark side, we all have difficult thoughts, feelings and impulses sometimes, its just part of being human.

- **Being proud of your experiences:** some people see their experience of psychosis as making them different from other people in a positive way. They view psychosis as a form of 'mental diversity' and think that it could mean they are more creative or insightful. There is a 'Mad Pride' movement which aims to create positive identities and rights for people with mental health problems. Many of the people who come to our groups say that the experience of psychosis has brought something positive in to their lives: greater empathy, a re-evaluation of priorities, a new career direction. We ask people if they could press a button to take their experience away, would they press it and many of them say 'no'.

- **Coming out:** some of the people who come to our group have also taken the brave step of starting to talk openly about their difficulties with families, friends, neighbours and colleagues. They've been worried about getting a bad reaction but actually they've found that people have been understanding, accepting and supportive. This has helped to reassure them people won't judge them and it has helped them to accept themselves too.

Research has shown that the best way to tackle stigma among people more generally is for them to get to know the people that they hold stereotypes about. This means that being open about your experiences can also make the world a better place, by changing people's attitudes. Some people, like James who we mentioned in chapter three, choose to tell their story publicly for this reason, getting involved with campaigns like 'Time to Change'. It's a way in which he feels he's turned his difficult experiences into something positive. You can find out more, and how you can get involved on their website: http://www.time-to-change.org.uk/

Melanie's experiences

When I have been honest about my mental health I have sometimes experienced stigma and lost a few friends but I think that 'those who mind don't matter and those who matter don't mind.'

When I have been told by people that something is not achievable or they feel that psychosis makes me incapable, I have questioned people's assumptions and continued to seek my own path.

Wanting to gain experience in mental health, I started as volunteer, and this helped me get onto the Occupational Therapy training course. When I qualified I got a job with the same manager who had recruited me as a volunteer, so my voluntary efforts paid off.

Since then I have tried to use my lived experience of mental health problems to my advantage when applying for work. For a number of years I have applied for jobs under the 'guaranteed interview' schemes available in many public sector organisations.

For mental health jobs I have been open and honest about experiencing psychosis. I see the interviews as a chance for me to shine but also for me to decide if I really want the job. I would not want to work somewhere that might discriminate against me. I feel I can do the job as well as anyone else, if not better, when I use empathy and my lived experience to inform me.

I am fortunate to work for one of an increasing number of mental health Trusts that seeks to employ people that have lived experience of mental health problems and then supports us to do the work.

There are many ways that I keep myself as well as possible and ensure I can continue to live the life I want. As well as eating five portions of fruit and vegetables a day I try to speak to someone (Connect), read something (Learn), go for a walk (Active), admire nature (Notice), and demonstrate friendly thoughtfulness (Give) each and every day.

Gratitude is another thing that is central to my recovery. Each night before I go to sleep I say a 'Thank You' prayer.

This helps to remind myself of even small good things that happen each day and train my brain to focus on the positive. Instead of writing them down in a Gratitude Diary I go over positive happenings in my head and thank God for each blessing. I believe this helps me to turn the tide towards thinking more positively generally.

I am lucky to have a few close and genuine friends. The friends that are peers who are also living with mental health problems have a way of making me feel accepted. When I talk about what makes me feel vulnerable I know they do not judge me. It is refreshing to talk to people who really understand what I have been through and make me I feel normal, and I hope I do the same for them.

I still find certain media stories and ignorance about mental health upsetting but I know many people from all different walks of life have to cope with society's discrimination. I think experiencing stigma makes people more empathic and sympathetic. I am a nicer person since having psychosis; I am kinder, less selfish, and more concerned about the happiness of others than I was before. My biggest struggle has turned out to be my greatest strength.

Section for reflection:

What activities could you do everyday to improve your wellbeing?

What are the opportunities in your area for you to connect with other people with similar experiences or use your experiences to give something back?

Has psychosis brought anything positive in to your life?

How would it feel to be open about your experiences, with people you know or as a way of tacking stigma?

Sources and resources

The ideas in this book come from lots of different places and are based on other people's work and experience. We've mentioned some, but not all, of them in the different chapters. So, we need to give the others credit too. Below is a complete list of the places we've taken our information from as well as some other places that you can look to find out more about how to understand and manage your experiences and live as well as possible.

Websites with resources to support mental health recovery and coping with psychosis

Coping with psychosis & voices

www.hearing-voices.org

www.intervoiceonline.org

www.rufusmay.com

Medication

www.comingoff.com

Recovery and wellbeing

www.workingtorecovery.co.uk

www.recoverydevon.co.uk

Other peer support

www.peerzone.info

www.madpride.org.uk

Spirituality

www.spiritualcrisisnetwork.org.uk

CBT resources

www.getselfhelp.co.uk

Books and articles to support mental health recovery and coping with psychosis

Recovery stories

Coleman, R. (1999). Recovery: An Alien Concept. Gloucester: Handsell Publishing

Cordle, H., Fradgely, J., Carson, J., Holloway, F. & Richards, P. (Eds) (2010). *Psychosis: Stories of Recovery and Hope.* London: Quay Books.

Deegan, P. (1996). Recovery and the Conspiracy of Hope. Presented at the Sixth Annual Mental Health Services Conference of Australia and New Zealand: Brisbane, Australia. Available to download from www.patdeegan.com/pat-deegan/lectures/conspiracy-of-hope

Chandler, R. & Hayward, M. (2009). Voicing Psychotic Experiences. Brighton: OLM-Pavilion

Romme, M., Escher, S., Dillon, J., Corstens, D. & Morris, M. (2009). *Living with Voices: 50 Stories of Recovery* : Ross-on-Wye: PCCS Books.

Mindfulness

Kabat-Zinn, J. (2004). Wherever You Go, There You Are: Mindfulness Meditation for Everyday Life. London: Piatkus Books.

Self-help for psychosis

Baker, P. (1998). The Voice Inside. P&P Press

Coleman, R. & Smith, M. (2005) (2nd ed). Working with Voices: Victim to Victor Workbook. P&P Press.

Coleman, R., Smith, M. & Good, J. (2001). Psychiatric First Aid. Gloucester: Handsell Publishing

Morrison, A. P., Renton, J., French, P. & Bentall, R. (2008). *Think You're Crazy, Think Again: A Resource Book for*

Cognitive Therapy for Psychosis. Hove: Routledge.

Turkington, D., Kingdon, D., Rathod, S., et al., (2009). *Back to life, Back to Normality*. Cambridge: CUP.

Making sense of psychosis

Bentall, R. (2004). *Madness Explained*. London: Penguin Books.
Read, J. & Sanders, P (2010). *A Straight-Talking Introduction to the Causes of Mental Health Problems*. PCCS Books

Medication

Holmes, G. & Hudson, M. (2003) Coming Off Medication, OpenMind, 123, 14-15. Available to download from www.psychologyintherealworld.co.uk
Moncreiff, J. (2009). A Straight Talking Introduction to Psychiatric Drugs. Ross-on-Wye: PCCS books.

Spiritual strategies

Psychic Self-Defence by Dion Fortune. Published by Red Wheel / Weiser
Handbook for the Urban Warrior by The Barefoot Doctor. Published by Piatkus Books.

Books and guides aimed at mental health workers and professionals

Chadwick, P. (2006). *Person-Based Cognitive Therapy for Distressing Psychosis.* Chichester: John Wiley.
Chadwick. P. K. (2008). Schizophrenia: The Positive Perspective: Explorations at the Outer Reaches of Human Experience. Hove: Routledge.

May R. (2004) Making sense of psychotic experiences and working towards recovery in Gleeson, J. and McGorry, P (Eds) *Psychological Interventions in Early Psychosis*. Chichester: Wiley.

Knight, T. (2009). *Beyond Belief: Alternative Ways of Working with Delusions, Obsessions and Unusual Experiences.* Shrewsbury: Peter Lehmann Publishing

Linehan, M.M. (1993). Skills Training Manual for Treating Borderline Personality Disorder. New York: Guilford Press.

Read, J. & Dillon, J. (2013). Models of Madness: Psychological, Social and Biological Approaches to Psychosis. London: Routledge.

Slade, M. (2009). One Hundred Ways to Support Recovery: A Guide for Mental Health Professionals. London: rethink. Available to download from www.rethink.org/about-us/commissioning-us/110-ways-to-support-recovery
Slade, M (2009). *Personal Recovery and Mental Illness: A Guide for Mental Health Professionals*. Cambridge: Cambridge University Press.

Research about psychosis, treatments, recovery and wellbeing

Appleby, L., Mortensen, P. B., Dunn, G., & Hiroeh, U. (2001). Death by homicide, suicide, and other unnatural causes in people with mental illness: a population-based study. *The Lancet*, 358, 2110-2112.

Beaven, V., Read, J. & Cartwright, C. (2011). The prevalence of voices hearers in the general population: A literature review. *Journal of Mental Health*, 20, pp 281-292.

Boyle, M. (2002). *Schizophrenia: A Scientific Delusion?* London: Routledge

Corrigan, P.W., Larson, J. E. & Rusch, N. (2009). Self-stigma and the "why try" effect: impact on life goals and evidence-based practices. *World Psychiatry*, 8, 75-81.

Deegan, P. E. (2005). The importance of personal medicine: A qualitative study of resilience in people with psychiatric disabilities. *Scandinavian Journal of Public Health*, 33 (66 suppl): 29–35

Dillon, J., Johnstone, L. & Longden, E. (2012). Trauma, Dissociation, Attachment & Neuroscience: A new paradigm for understanding severe mental distress. *The Journal of Critical Psychology, Counselling and Psychotherapy*, 12, pp 145-155.

Freeman, D. (2007). Suspicious minds: The psychology of paranoid delusions. *Clinical Psychology Review*, 27, pp 425-427.

Ellet, L., Lopes, B. & Chadwick, P. (2003). Paranoia in a non-clinical population of college students. *Journal of Nervous and Mental Disease*, 191, pp 425-30.

Holmes, T.H. & Rahe, R. H. (1967). "The Social Readjustment Rating Scale". *Journal of Psychosomatic Research* 11, 213–8.

Meehan, T., Stedman, T. & Wallace, J. (2011). Consumer Strategies for Coping With Antipsychotic Medication Side Effects. *Australasian Psychiatry*, 19, pp 74-77.

Morrison, A.P, Hutton, P., Shiers, D. & Turkington, D. (2012) Antipsychotics: is it time to introduce patient choice? *The British Journal of Psychiatry 201, 83–84.*

New Economics Foundation (2008). *Foresight Mental Capital and Wellbeing Project: Making the Most of Ourselves in the 21st Century*. London: The Government Office for Science.

Pilgrim, D. & Rogers, A. (2003). Mental disorder and violence: An empirical picture in context. *Journal of Mental Health*, 12. 7-18.

Romme, M. & Escher, S. (1993) *Accepting Voices*. Mind Publications, London.

Zubin, J. and Spring, B. (1977) Vulnerability: A New View on Schizophrenia *Journal of Abnormal Psychology* 86, 103-126